Specialist Training in:

SEXUALLY TRANSMITTED INFECTIONS AND HIV

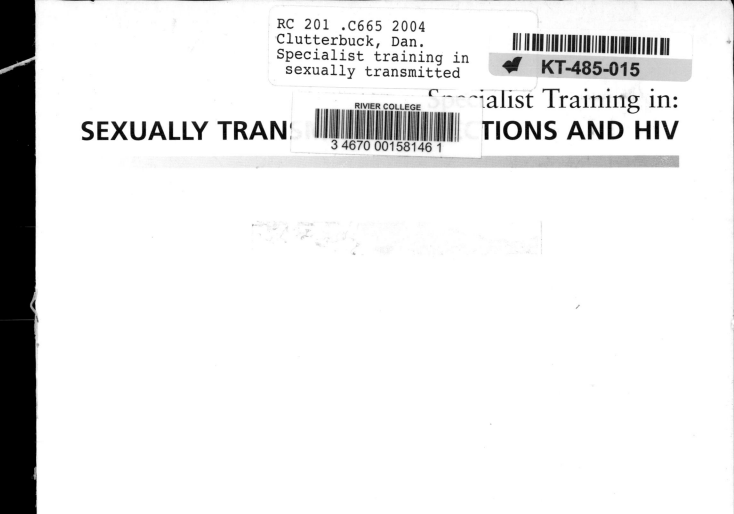

Commissioning Editor: Timothy Horne
Project Development Manager: Clive Hewat
Project Manager: Nancy Arnott
Designer: George Ajayi

Specialist Training in:
SEXUALLY TRANSMITTED INFECTIONS AND HIV

Dan Clutterbuck BSc MBChB MRCP MRCGP DFFP

Consultant G.U.M. Physician, Lothian University Hospitals, Edinburgh, UK

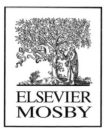

Edinburgh London New York Oxford Philadelphia St Louis Sydney Toronto 2004

ELSEVIER
MOSBY

First published 2004

ISBN 0723432848

British Library Cataloguing in Publication Data
A catalogue record for this book is available from the British Library

Library of Congress Cataloging in Publication Data
A catalog record for this book is available from the Library of Congress

Notice
Medical knowledge is constantly changing. Standard safety precautions must be followed, but as new research and clinical experience broaden our knowledge, changes in treatment and drug therapy may become necessary or appropriate. Readers are advised to check the most current product information provided by the manufacturer of each drug to be administered to verify the recommended dose, the method and duration of administration, and contraindications. It is the responsibility of the practitioner, relying on experience and knowledge of the patient, to determine dosages and the best treatment for each individual patient. Neither the Publisher nor the author assumes any liability for any injury and/or damage to persons or property arising from this publication.
The Publisher

ELSEVIER your source for books,
journals and multimedia
in the health sciences

www.elsevierhealth.com

The
publisher's
policy is to use
**paper manufactured
from sustainable forests**

Printed in China

Preface

This book is intended for those new to the management of sexually transmitted infections and HIV. It should serve professionals in the first few months of a career in the specialty of genitourinary medicine as a first port-of-call for a quick review during a busy clinic. I've also tried to make it useable in all the settings I've experienced – including family planning clinics and general practice as well as the teaching hospital GUM department and rural district general hospital – and by medical and non-medical professionals. Hence the recommendations for the diagnosis and management of common conditions are sufficiently detailed to make it useful where it is the only text available to the non-specialist involved in STI care. The commonest problems and those posing the greatest challenge to those new to the field, such as chlamydial infection and the management of bloodborne virus exposure, are covered in the greatest detail. History taking, information for patients and specific treatment recommendations form the bulk of the text, although brief details of pathogenesis and the management of rarer conditions are included. Much of the core information is presented as tables with illustrations, flow diagrams and other aids to diagnosis and management. The chapters on HIV infection concentrate on the outpatient management in the specialist clinic or in general practice, with the emphasis on holistic care and the use of antiretroviral therapy.

Dan Clutterbuck
Edinburgh 2004

Acknowledgements

I am particularly indebted to my colleague and mentor Dr Sandy McMillan who suggested the project and has provided advice and encouragement throughout. I owe thanks to several others: my colleagues at the Royal Infirmary of Edinburgh: Dr Gordon Scott, Dr Carolyn Thompson, Dr Jaqueline Paterson and Dr Kaveh Manavi read and commented on chapters. The nurses and health advisers I have worked with at the Victoria Hospital, Kirkcaldy and at Borders Sexual Health, Melrose 'test ran' many of the chapters as tutorials and teaching materials, providing invaluable input. Dr Hugh Young provided data from the Scottish Neisseria Gonorrhoeae Reference Laboratory and the Chlamydia Laboratory, University of Edinburgh Medical School. Drs McMillan and Scott kindly permitted the use of photographs from their book. (Figures 1.1, 3.1, 3.2, 3.3, 3.4, 4.1, 5.1, 5.2, 6.1, 6.2, 6.3, 7.1, 7.2, 10.1 and 10.2 reprinted from McMillan and Scott – *Sexually Transmitted Infections – Colour Guide 2e*, Copyright 2000, with permission from Elsevier.) Dr Mark Pakianathan and colleagues of The Courtyard Clinic, St. Georges Hospital, London; Dr Gillian Dean of Essex County Hospital, Brighton; Dr Philip Welsby of the Western General Hospital, Edinburgh and Dr Paddy Gibb of the Department of Medical Microbiology, University of Edinburgh provided photographs from their collections. Cath Cassidy, of Healthy Respect, Lothian Health Board, provided photographs of chlamydia testing kits. Alan Wilson of the Infectious Diseases Unit, Western General Hospital, Edinburgh, spent considerable time transferring slides to CD Rom for the project and Ann Chiswick of the same department obtained the photographs of antiretroviral drugs. I'm especially grateful to Dr John White for arranging access to the collection bequeathed to the Australasian College of Sexual Health Physicians by the widow of the late Dr Don Jacobs. The college President, Dr David Bradford, generously gave his permission to use the images. Finally, thanks to my partner Tim for his support.

D.C.

Contents

Sexually transmitted infections in the sexual health consultation

THE CONSULTATION

The diagnosis and treatment of people with sexually transmitted infection (STI) and the management of those who are concerned about the possibility of infection depends upon the quality of the initial consultation. The core of this consultation is the sexual history; so sexual history taking is described in considerable detail here. In the UK, for most of the twentieth century, genitourinary medicine (GUM) clinics provided care for those with STIs. As the number of STIs diagnosed in GUM increases (Fig. 1.1), they are also frequently diagnosed in settings other than GUM clinics (Fig. 1.2). Consequently, the sexual history must be discussed by practitioners from diverse backgrounds in the course of their routine work (Box 1.1). A relaxed, non-judgemental approach to discussing sex and STIs makes all such consultations much easier, but the development of a systematic approach to questioning is vital.

Concerns about confidentiality are central to health-care practice and are heightened when STIs are involved. Young people are disproportionately affected by STIs and issues relating to consent and confidentiality in younger teenagers must be considered. A comprehensive sexual history is crucial in directing clinical examination and collection of the appropriate microbiological specimens (see pp. 14–26), as well as for the provision of counselling and information on STIs.

SEXUAL-HISTORY TAKING

Background

In dedicated facilities such as the GUM clinic, questions relating to STIs may be easy to introduce. Where the agenda is more general, introducing such questions can be more difficult.

Medical history taking outside the GU field has traditionally avoided questions relating to STI symptoms, same-sex partners, psychosexual problems and the risk of blood-borne viruses.

Sexual health has been equated with 'women's health', leaving men entirely out of the equation. Men make up half or more of attendees to many GUM services.

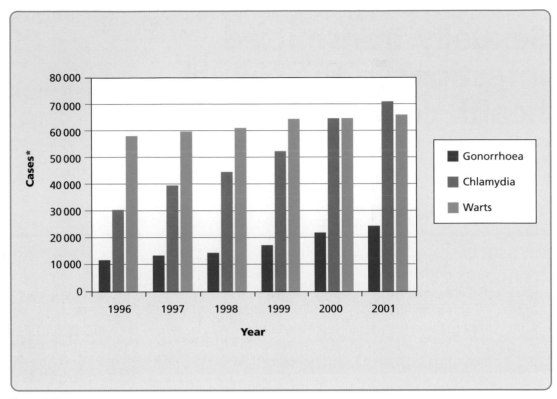

Figure 1.1
Cases of three selected common STI diagnoses 1996–2001.
*Number of cases of uncomplicated gonorrhoea, chlamydial infection and first episode warts, GUM clinics, England, Wales and Northern Ireland, 1996–2001.
(Data from PHLS, DHSS & PS and the Scottish ISD (D)5 Collaborative Group, 2002.)

Those new to sexual health, or whose field has changed to include STIs may have to relearn history taking in order to address these issues appropriately.

Discussion of 'difficult' topics may be eased by allowing more time. As this luxury is rarely available, we need techniques to facilitate efficient assessment of complex and delicate problems.

The attributes of good sexual history taking are detailed in Box 1.2.

Learning how

A flexible and less formal approach is needed for work in sexual health. If you feel less comfortable outside the 'traditional' consultation, don't despair – the skills required can be learned, though not solely from a book. Consider a shared clinic with a mentor (perhaps seeing alternate patients) or, if facilities are available, video or audiotape analysis of consultation skills to improve practice. The schema described here provides a starting point.

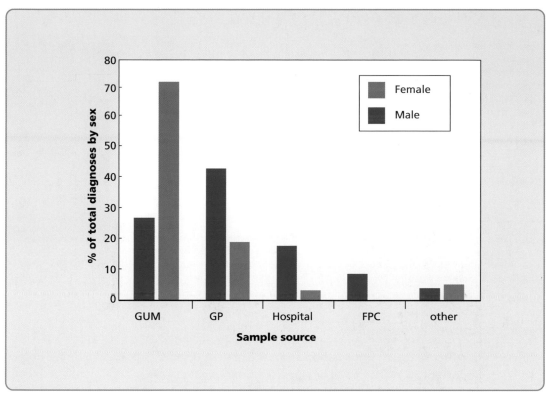

Figure 1.2
Positive tests for *Chlamydia trachomatis* by sample source, Lothian, 2002. Source of 2322 positive tests in Lothian, South-East Scotland.
(Data courtesy of Chlamydia laboratory, Dept of Medical Microbiology, University of Edinburgh Medical School.)

Box 1.1: Consultations where sexually transmitted infections may be discussed

Symptomatic patients
Patients aware that their presenting symptoms may be due to STI
Patients unaware that their presenting symptoms may be due to STI
Patients presenting with atypical symptoms perceived as being due to STI (common, often related to anxieties about a sexual contact)
Victims of rape and sexual assault

Asymptomatic patients
Patients requesting prophylactic STI screening (e.g. before a new relationship)
Patients with recent sexual contacts at risk of STI
Patients with serological or microbiological evidence of STI found on screening (e.g. blood donors)
Opportunistic testing for STI:
– cervical smear
– termination clinic
– post coital contraception
– antenatal clinic.
Victims of rape and sexual assault

Box 1.2: Good sexual history taking

- Effective
- Efficient
- Inoffensive
- Inclusive
- Non-judgemental
- Permission giving
- Avoids labelling
- Avoids gender laden language

Box 1.3: Making the right start

- Welcome the patient
- Collect the patient from a waiting room
- Look at the patient and smile (even if it is the 50th patient of the day). Introduce yourself. Wear a name badge
- Sit at about 90° to the patient, across the corner of the desk if there is one
- Adopt an open posture

Basic communication skills

Eliciting sensitive information from the patient depends upon developing rapport, so it's important to make the right start (see Box 1.3, Fig. 1.3).

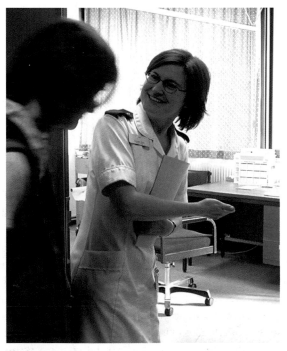

Figure 1.3
Making the right start

Many patients do not wish to meet your eye directly when discussing sexual matters, so respect this, but give plenty of opportunity for brief eye contact or a nod of encouragement. Make use of silence to give the patient time to discuss things they may never have discussed before. When you suspect that there is an unexpressed concern, saying so may prompt disclosure. Use reflection and summarize to clarify detail (Clinical notes below). It's unusual not to be embarrassed occasionally, but the experience can be constructive (see Box 1.4).

Box 1.4: On embarrassment

Virtually everyone is occasionally caught out by something brought up in a consultation. You may frequently be embarrassed in the early days of talking about sexual health. It is possible to brazen out an episode of red-faced stammering, but often helpful to acknowledge what has happened. Admitting your own discomfort can be a great leveller and can improve the consultation:

I've embarrassed us both by asking that question...but I'd really like you to tell me more about it

I could have phrased that better...how about you just tell me what happened?

I wasn't really expecting you to say that – but please carry on

---

Clinical notes: history taking

Reflection:

Patient: I just feel dirty
Doctor: Dirty...?
Patient: Like I might have caught something
Doctor: Something like...?
Patient: Well I don't know, like AIDS or something.

Summarizing:
So, it was about 2 weeks after you split up with your regular partner that you had sex with the guy in Manchester, and about 1 week later that you noticed the discharge...

A prompt:
I get the feeling that there is something you are finding hard to say...

Language

Use simple, clear language. Basic anatomical terms are appropriate for most patients, but make sure it is clear to you both what is being discussed. Describe things simply, in detail, and in the vernacular. Conversely, be cautious of introducing vague sexual colloquialisms or offensive slang words *unless introduced by the patient*. Usually you may let the patient set the tone of language to be used. Gently suggesting the appropriate street word is often enough to 'give permission' for its use. Use the patient's own language, but try to avoid repeating (and thereby sanctioning) pejorative phrases. Patients may be flippant – often to disguise nervousness. It is dangerous to succumb to the temptation to be flippant oneself in such circumstances. Smile, but try to steer the patient back to a basic account of the problem. The sexual history should extend only as far as is required to deal with the patient's physical and emotional problems. Although it's often necessary to talk in detail about intimate details of patients' lives, beware of lapsing into voyeurism.

Case history

Sabrina (19 years of age) mentioned lower abdominal pain when attending for a repeat oral contraceptive prescription. Some questions the doctor used in deciding to test for STIs were:

- 'Tell me more about the pain'
- 'Had you any thoughts about what the pain might be?'
- 'Do you have a partner just now?'
- 'When did you last have sex, any sort of sex?'
- 'Does having sex affect the pain?'
- 'Is that outside, on the lips of your vagina, or deep inside?'

Foreign language

Non-English-speaking patients may arrive with a translator who may be a partner, friend or a child. Unless the problem is of real urgency, try to arrange a return visit with a professional translator. Translation services are increasingly available by phone. Ask the switchboard at the nearest major hospital about local services, or in the UK try Language Line Limited (0800 169 2879) or EITI Limited (0870 701 2020), to find out whether they have an arrangement with your local health provider.

Good translators may be able to give you valuable insights regarding cultural attitudes to sex and relationships. However, even with professional translators there can be problems:

- In small ethnic communities the patient may know the translator
- Not all translators are comfortable discussing sexual matters. Make the translation service aware that sex will be discussed
- Patients may be unhappy discussing sexual matters in the presence of someone from their own culture of the opposite sex.

It is sometimes uncomfortable to reflect after the consultation on whether the standards of confidentiality offered in the clinic to a non-English-speaking patient are the same as those offered to an English speaker.

Introducing questions about STIs in other consultations

Aim to get to the direct question, 'When did you last have sex?', as sensitively and efficiently as possible (Box 1.5). It can be difficult to introduce the question when the consultation is not initially related to sexual matters. Different openers are possible in different circumstances:

- Where symptoms suggest possible STI. Openers may occur when discussing abdominal or pelvic pain – 'Does anything else make the pain worse?' and 'Does having sex affect the pain?'; when taking a menstrual history – 'Is there any chance you could be pregnant?' and 'When did you last have sex?'; or when discussing an itch or discharge – 'Do you think there's any chance that this could be a sexually transmitted infection?'.

> **Box 1.5: Asking about sexual intercourse**
>
> **'When did you last have sex, any sort of sex?':**
>
> - Avoids assumptions regarding partner(s), gender, timing, sexual acts
> - Allows questions relating to a partner without attaching value laden labels (e.g. 'was that with a man?' rather than 'are you a homosexual?')
> - Avoids the assumption of monogamy
> - Avoids the assumption that all partners are of the same gender

- Where concerns about STI are suspected. Discussions about low mood, relationship problems, or undisclosed anxiety may suggest an opener – 'Has this affected your sex life?'.
- When targeting screening for infections. The question may be introduced at a routine cervical smear appointment – 'How's sex?' or 'How's your sex life?'.
- Questions can be introduced 'out of the blue' – 'Who is at home with you?', 'Do you have a partner?', 'Are you living on your own?', or 'Is it okay if I ask you about your sex life?'.

Clinical notes: history taking

Some questions and phrases to avoid:

- 'Are you married?'
- 'Are you married yet?'
- 'Have you had any questionable consorts?'
- 'I'm sorry to ask you this but...'
- 'There's no need to be embarrassed, but...'
- 'As a routine part of your medical care, I need to ask you some questions about your sexual health.'
- Any other preamble that says to the patient 'I'm embarrassed about this, so you should be too.'

A SCHEMA FOR THE STI HISTORY

Although there are no rules for taking a sexual medical history, it can be helpful to have a schema to fall back on. Once you are comfortable with taking a structured history, it becomes much easier to talk freely around the problem, obtaining all the information required, in a much less formal manner.

Communication style is a very personal aspect of practice and some of the phrasing suggested here may not suit you. The approach can be adapted over time to suit your own style and also the values and colloquialisms of the population you serve.

The history

'How can I help?' is as good an opener as any. Train yourself to allow at least a minute of merely nodding, prompting and reflecting words and phrases, which will often reveal the problem in its entirety. You will encounter patients who have taken months or years to get to the stage of expressing concerns verbally – don't underestimate the importance of that first minute. Avoid any distraction (such as logging a patient in on a computer) that interrupts the initial flow of the consultation.

In symptomatic patients ask about details of the presenting problem, starting with open, then closed questions. Specific questions relating to pain, discharge and so on are detailed in the appropriate chapters.

Ask about the timescale of the problem. If the problem is recent and the patient has not mentioned any triggers try the following prompt:

Did anything happen at the start of this problem that you thought may have caused it?

If the problem is longstanding, the following may help produce more information:

What made you come to see us just now – have things got worse, or changed?

Probably the very best question in any history, which is familiar to generations of GPs, is: 'Have you had any thoughts yourself about what might be going on?' This may elicit answers such as, 'Well, my mate said there's this Chlamyddy thing...'

Asymptomatic patients may simply ask for a 'full check' or 'tests for infections'. These requests sometimes come out of the blue, but much more often are precipitated by an event worth knowing about. It is always worth asking, 'Any reason why that has come up just now?'

Partners

Asking 'Are you married?' or something similar conveys an assumption of monogamous heterosexuality. It isn't enough to be non-judgemental, you may have to overcome patients' negative expectations of you as an 'authority figure'. The use of the term 'partner' is neutral and universally applicable. Even if a partner has been mentioned, it is useful to review things. Don't assume that all partners will be of the same gender.

'Do you have a sexual partner (at the moment/just now)?' is useful, particularly when dealing with young people who may not have had a sexual partner.

'When did you last have sex?' is more direct. It is useful to add 'any sort of sex' to attempt to avoid confusion over what constitutes sex (see Box 1.5).

Many hours have been spent developing definitions of 'casual' and 'regular' partners for questionnaires in behavioural research. It is probably best to let patients define these for themselves, asking more specific questions where necessary. Often, if you have put the patient at ease and he or she has decided that you are 'OK', you may well get all of these details without asking specifically.

If you really don't want to ask about the partner's gender, the answer to the question 'Has your partner had any symptoms?' will usually require the use of a personal pronoun indicating gender. It's not acceptable to avoid asking about a partner's gender just because, for example, the patient is a male construction worker.

Sexual activities

Talking about specific acts seems to be 'another level' of taboo, causing embarrassment to patients who may otherwise speak quite freely about sexual matters. It therefore requires particular care.

Oral sex

The terms cunnilingus and fellatio just aren't used. Most people understand the phrases 'oral sex' and 'go down on' as in 'did you go down on her or did she go down on you?'. Sometimes a more straightforward anatomical description is better.

Anal sex

Unprotected anal sex is a risk factor for HIV in men who have sex with men, as well as in heterosexual women (in studies 5–20% of heterosexual women report having had anal sex). Don't assume that sex between men means anal sex and avoid using terms such as 'active' and 'passive' or 'top' and 'bottom'. Possible approaches include, 'Did you penetrate him or did he penetrate you?', or 'Do you give or take or both?'. Many gay men will be quite happy with the use of the vernacular 'fuck' to describe anal sex, but as with other slang words, it is safest to wait until the patient introduces them.

Rimming

Oro-anal sexual contact ('rimming') may transmit gastrointestinal pathogens such as *Giardia intestinalis* in men who have sex with men. The phrase is likely to be familiar to most men who do it, but a simple anatomical description is an alternative.

Fisting

Brachioproctic eroticism or brachiovaginal eroticism: insertion of several fingers, the cupped hand or the forearm into the rectum or vagina. It is likely to involve significant superficial trauma to the rectal or vaginal mucosa and is, therefore, potentially a risk factor for HIV transmission, particularly when followed by peno-vaginal or peno-anal intercourse.

Travel

It is important to ask in which part of the world sex took place and to ask the nationality of sexual contacts. Travellers, including tourists and 'gap-year' travellers are at increased risk of STI. Don't assume that sex abroad will have been with a partner of local origin.

Protection and contraception

Asking about the use of barrier protection can be difficult. If you ask, 'Did you use a condom?', most people will say 'Yes'. Be aware that many patients will have used a condom for part of the time, such as just before ejaculation, or may have removed the condom after ejaculation.

Other partners

One particularly effective phrase is, 'When did you last have sex with a partner other than that one?' (see Box 1.6). 'When did you last have sex with anyone else?' is simpler, but occasionally upsets those in regular monogamous relationships who take it to mean you assume infidelity. If there are many partners, you could simply ask, 'How many others in the last 3 months?'.

Box 1.6: Asking about other partners

'When did you last have sex with a partner other than that one?'

- Allows the patient to disclose sex with a partner prior to a current relationship, or whilst in a current relationship
- Allows patients to discuss multiple regular partners
- Implies no assumption of infidelity in a regular relationship
- Implies no assumption of serial monogamy (as in 'prior to that one')

Other details

You should also ask about:

- past medical history, including STIs
- a history of hepatitis or hepatitis vaccination
- drug intake (prescribed and recreational), in particular antimicrobials taken in the last month
- adverse reactions to drugs
- a menstrual history in women
- an obstetric history in women
- cervical smears in women.

Social factors, self-esteem and psychological well-being are intimately related to sexual health – particularly to the risk of recurrent STI or unwanted pregnancy. A full assessment should, ideally, be part of every sexual health consultation. Time pressures rarely allow this, but try to stay alert to those cases where a more detailed exploration is necessary. Box 1.7 shows a summary of the sexual history.

CONFIDENTIALITY, CONSENT AND YOUNG PEOPLE

CONFIDENTIALITY

General medical confidentiality

General medical confidentiality in the UK is a common law duty (that is it is not defined by specific legislation, but by judgements in previous legal cases).

The duty of confidentiality to the patient is absolute except in certain very specific circumstances, such as when another individual is placed at risk of death or serious harm, or in child-protection cases. These circumstances occasionally arise in sexual health when an individual known to have HIV infection withholds this information from a partner with whom he or she continues to have unprotected sex.

The duty of confidentiality extends beyond death.

Box 1.7: Summary of the sexual history

Subject	Question	Notes and alternatives
Opening question	'How can I help?'	Allow at least 1 minute Patient's agenda Use prompts, reflection
Questions about symptoms	'Tell me more about that' '... any pain?'	Open questions at first Then closed questions
Timescale	'Did anything happen at the start of this problem that you thought may have caused it?'	'What did you think was going on?'
	'What made you come to see us just now – have things got worse, or changed?'	
Partners	'Do you have a partner?'	
	'Is (was) that a casual partner or a regular partner?' or	'Was that a relationship or just a one off?'
	'Is (was) that a new partner?	'... a regular thing or just once?'
	'How long have you been with that partner?'	
Last sexual contact	'When did you last have sex...any sex?' 'Is your partner male or female?' or 'was that with a man or a woman?' (or 'is that a male partner?' or 'is that a female partner?' if you feel you don't want to hedge your bets)	'... a guy or a girl?'
	'Where is she from?'	'Is (was) that a man from the UK?'
Sexual activities	'Oral sex, anal sex, both or neither?' 'Did you penetrate him or did he penetrate you?'	
Other partners	'When did you last have sex with a partner other than that one – any other partner, any other sex?'	'When did you last have sex with anyone else?'
Condom use	'Did you use condoms with (either, any) of those partners?' '– just some of the time or all the time?'	'Do you ever use condoms?' 'When did you last have sex without a condom?'

Confidentiality in STI management

In the UK, confidentiality in the management of people treated for STIs, is defined by statute in the Venereal Diseases Acts of 1917 and 1921 and subsequent NHS regulations.

Patient notes in GUM clinics are kept separately from other hospital notes. Patients are required to give only minimal information at registration (e.g. a first name and date of birth).

General practitioners are not usually routinely informed of a patient's attendance at a GUM clinic unless the patient is initially referred by letter.

If it is in the patient's interest for another health-care worker to be informed, the patient's consent to disclosure must be sought.

Practicalities

Practice a 'need to know' policy. Information should be shared only with those directly involved with the care of the patient.

All clinics should have soundproof consulting rooms and offices to allow discussion in complete privacy. In practice this is not always the case. Many GUM and other clinics operate in poor accommodation with substandard facilities. Don't allow this to compromise confidentiality.

Confidentiality and sexual contacts

Partner notification, or contact tracing, involves identifying, counselling and screening the sexual partners of those with STIs in order to break the chain of transmission. The routes of notification are:

1. Patient referral: the index patient (the one with infection) tells the partner of the need to attend a clinic. This may involve a 'contact slip' (see Fig. 1.4), a note recording the index patient's clinic number, the clinic name and a code representing the infection treated.
2. Provider referral: the index patient gives the health-care worker information, such as name and address of sexual partner(s). The health worker contacts the partner(s) independently by phone, letter, or occasionally in person.
3. Conditional referral: the patient agrees to contact sexual partners, but agrees to refer the matter to the clinic or health-care worker if no contact has been made after an agreed time period has elapsed.

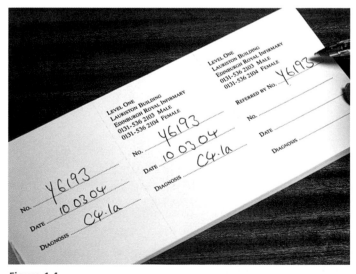

Figure 1.4
Completing a contact slip

Effective partner notification is complex and specialized work usually undertaken by professional health advisers. Other health-care workers working in sexual health will encounter patients who attend as contacts of those with infection. Maintaining confidentiality in these cases can be challenging. In such consultations:

- The index patient must not be identified. The health worker must not confirm the identity of the index, even when raised by the patient. Obviously, in those patients with only one sexual partner, it may be impossible to avoid identification.
- The patient may know the identity of the index, if patient referral has taken place. However, all other information relating to the index remains confidential.
- A good working principle is to say nothing about the index, including the diagnosis, unless first raised by the patient. Start by establishing exactly what the contact has been told.

CONSENT AND CONFIDENTIALITY IN THOSE UNDER 16

Many sexual health consultations will take place with people under the age of 16. Fears regarding confidentiality are a significant barrier to young people seeking contraceptive and other sexual health advice. Make it a priority to familiarize yourself with local and national policies on consent, confidentiality and child-protection guidelines. A few pointers applicable to the UK are included here.

Consent and those under 16

In England and Wales the law relating to consent for those under 16 was established by the Law Lords ruling on the Gillick case, in Scotland it was established by the Age of Legal Capacity Act, 1991.

Any competent young person, regardless of age, can independently seek medical advice and give valid consent to treatment.

Competency reflects the young person's ability to understand the choices available and their possible consequences. So called 'Gillick competence' applies to people under 16 attending for contraceptive advice, but is helpful in all sexual health consultations. In essence, you should:

- ensure that the patient understands the risks and benefits of the treatment or advice given
- discuss the value of parental support – a doctor is legally obliged to do this. Young people should be encouraged to inform parents, and reasons for not doing so should be explored, but they should be made aware that their confidentiality would be respected should they choose not to do so
- take into account whether the person is likely to have sexual intercourse without contraception
- assess whether the person's physical or mental health, or both, are likely to suffer if the person does not receive contraceptive advice or supplies
- consider whether the patient's best interests are served by the provision of contraception without parental consent.

Confidentiality and those under 16

The duty of confidentiality owed to a person under 16 is the same as that for any other person.

You have no legal obligation to report criminal conduct except for terrorist offences or road traffic offences.

It is illegal for people under the age of 16 to have sex. For most doctors in most cases there is no question of reporting underage sex to the Police or Social Work departments. In almost every case it is possible to respect the right of absolute confidentiality. However, extremely difficult decisions may be faced in particular circumstances:

- When there is a question of abuse, such as evidence of physical harm or allegation or suspicion of incest
- When the patient is under the age of consent and the partner is significantly older
- When coercion or financial exploitation is suspected
- When there is doubt about the ability to give consent – for example, with young patients (the law considers a girl under the age of 12 unable to give consent) or with those with learning disabilities.

In these cases you may not be able to guarantee confidentiality. It is sometimes useful to discuss both your commitment to confidentiality and the limits of that confidentiality early in the consultation. If there is thought to be immediate risk to the individual or another (for example, a sibling), it may be necessary to contact child-protection agencies. Most areas have a senior social worker who can be contacted to discuss details of cases without disclosing the identity of the individual. If confidentiality is to be broken it must be discussed honestly with the patient and in detail with senior colleagues. Consider the law, the individual's interest, the public interest and professional duty.

Young people hear about services by word of mouth. Potential users of the service involved are likely to find out about any breach of confidentiality.

PHYSICAL EXAMINATION AND SPECIMEN COLLECTION

PATIENTS, DIGNITY AND EXAMINATION

Young men are often completely unfamiliar with dealing with medical services and women below the age of first cervical screening may not previously have had an internal or speculum examination. The examination should be explained in detail to these patients before they undress. It may be worth cutting short history taking as soon as it is clear what microbiological samples will be required and proceeding to examination, allowing the patient to relax and talk more freely afterwards. Allow patients to undress and prepare themselves before you enter an examination area or cubicle. (The experience of undressing whilst observed is even more intimate and personal than that of being seen unclothed). The use of a chaperone is mandatory for male health-care workers with female patients and is desirable in all cases.

Full physical examination can be combined with the taking of routine specimens. Many doctors confine routine examination to the genital area unless the history suggests that full examination is necessary. Although this is adequate in asymptomatic patients, adding routine examination of the skin, mouth (see Fig. 1.5) and abdomen takes only a few extra seconds and will improve your diagnostic skills while training. It is also a non-threatening way in which to place your hands on the patient whilst maintaining conversation and eye contact, before examining the genitals.

Systemic examination of all patients

Skin. Look for rash or evidence of excoriation (Figs 1.6, 1.7). Include the elbows, the webs of the fingers and the plantar aspect of the wrists.

Mouth. Look for erosions, ulcers, chancre, oral hairy leukoplakia or candidiasis.

Neck. Palpate for lymphadenopathy, checking axillary nodes if neck nodes are palpable.

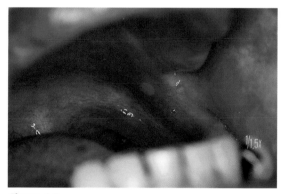

Figure 1.5
Oral ulceration in Behçet's disease

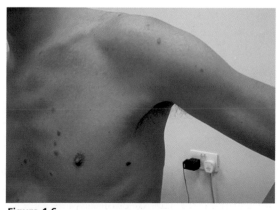

Figure 1.6
Kaposi's sarcoma seen in a patient requesting tests for STIs

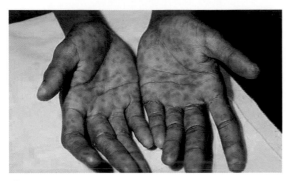

Figure 1.7
Rash of secondary syphilis on the palms

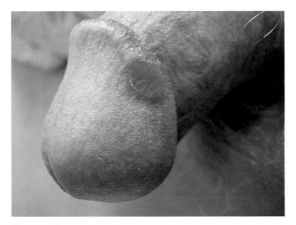

Figure 1.8
Psoriasis of the glans penis

Abdomen. Palpate for evidence of hepatosplenomegaly (HIV, syphilis) or for distension or tenderness of the bladder in men with dysuria.

Inguinal lymph nodes. Palpate, noting size, consistency and any tenderness.

Skin of the genital area (Fig. 1.8). Check for the presence of *Pthirus pubis* (crab lice) in the pubic hair and the hair on the abdomen and thighs. Look for genital warts, molluscum contagiosum, scaling or erythema indicating possible fungal infection over the pubis, groins and genitalia. A hand lens is sometimes useful when examining small skin lesions or searching for evidence of crab lice.

ROUTINE EXAMINATION AND SPECIMEN COLLECTION IN MEN

Examination procedure

Expose at least the lower abdomen and the genitalia, with the trousers lowered to the knees.

Take samples for the identification of *Neisseria gonorrhoeae* from the pharynx (Box 1.8) in:

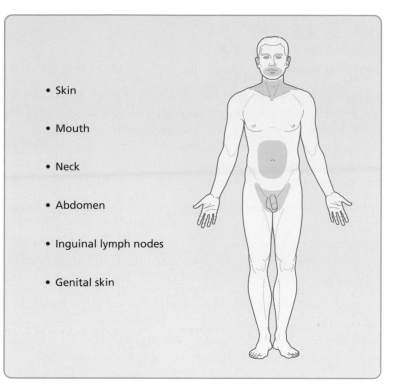

- Skin

- Mouth

- Neck

- Abdomen

- Inguinal lymph nodes

- Genital skin

Examination Box 1.1: Systemic examination in STI care

Box 1.8: Microbiological specimens in men

Pharynx
Use a cotton-tipped swab to sample material from both tonsils and tonsillar fossae, sweeping the swab quickly over the soft palate and uvula. Plate direct onto culture medium or into charcoal medium for later plating for culture for *N. gonorrhoeae* (see Ch. 4).

Urethra
Gently part the urethral meatus, applying slight traction to extend the penis. Insert a plastic loop into the meatus, directing it towards the dorsal aspect of the penis. Sample material (Fig. 1.13) from the distal 2 cm of the urethra by applying gentle lateral pressure on withdrawing the loop. In men with symptoms suggestive of urethritis but no obvious discharge, it may be worthwhile 'stripping' the urethra – applying finger pressure from the perineum to the tip of the penis to express discharge for sampling.

In ALL men
Urethral sample for testing for *N. gonorrhoeae*. Take a 20 ml sample of first voided urine for DNA amplification or obtain material from the distal 2–4 cm of the urethra using a sterile cotton-tipped ENT swab for detection of *C. trachomatis*.

If required
Smear a sample of material on a glass slide for Gram staining and microscopy for identification of *N. gonorrhoeae* and diagnosis of non-gonococcal urethritis (NGU) (either immediately, or air dried and sent with the patient to a clinic). A single sample is usually sufficient for both Gram stained smear and inoculation of a culture plate.

Rectum
In all men who have sex with men. Use a cotton wool swab (dry, or moistened with sterile saline) passed about 3 cm into the anal canal to obtain a sample from the anal canal and the terminal rectum for culture for *N. gonorrhoeae*. Take a second sample for testing for *C. trachomatis* infection.

In those with symptoms or signs of rectal infection. Under direct vision at proctoscopy, take a sample using a plastic loop from any area of pus or mucopus for Gram staining and microscopy for *N. gonorrhoeae*. In men with rectal symptoms in whom inflammation is seen on proctoscopy, take a further sample for testing for herpes simplex virus infection and ask the patient to provide a stool sample for examination for bacteria and protozoa.

- ALL men who have sex with men
- Heterosexual men who are contacts of gonorrhoea
- Heterosexual men who have Gram-negative intracellular diplococci on urethral smear.

Penis. Examine for dermatoses. Retract the foreskin fully, if present, and check for inflammation of the glans (balanitis) or foreskin (posthitis). Warts, erosions, ulcers, chancre and occasionally tumours may be seen on the glans or inner aspect of the foreskin. Note the presence of congenital abnormalities such as hypospadias, and common anatomical features such as prominent coronal papillae (Figs 1.9, 1.10), occasionally perceived as abnormal by patients.

Urethral meatus. Examine for presence of discharge (Fig. 1.11), ulcers, inflammation or intrameatal warts. If discharge covers the glans, this may be removed with a swab. Microbiological specimens for identification of *N. gonorrhoeae* and *Chlamydia trachomatis* are required in all men (Box 1.8). A sample for Gram-stain microscopy is also required in men with:

- Contact of non-specific urethritis (NSU)/non-specific genital infection (NSGI)/pelvic inflammatory disease (PID)/gonorrhoea
- Symptoms of urethritis
- Evidence of urethral discharge or inflammation on urethral examination.

Scrotum. Examine for erythema or rash. Tinea cruris commonly affects the scrotum and the skin of the adjacent thigh. Sebaceous cysts may be seen – they need no intervention. Palpate the scrotum, confirming the presence of two approximately equal sized testes, separate epididymes and the absence of any unusual enlargement, mass or tenderness. Many young men in the sexual health clinic will not have been examined since childhood, and it is usual to find small cysts in the epididymis or a testicular varicocoele (commoner on the left) that have not previously been noted. Less commonly, no testis can be felt in one side of the scrotum and the patient is unable to confirm that it descends, in which

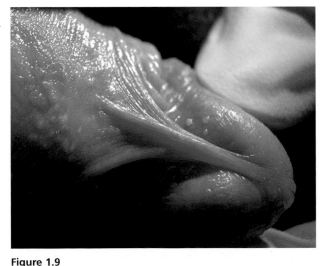

Figure 1.9
Coronal papillae

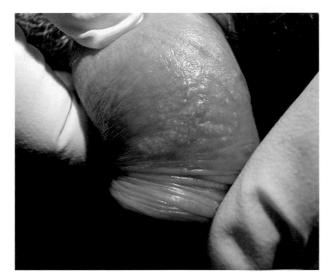

Figure 1.10
Sebaceous glands

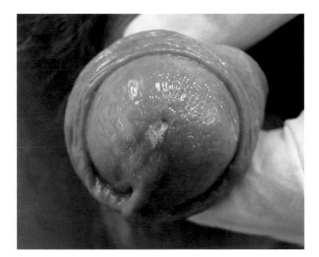

Figure 1.11
Discharge at the urethral meatus

case surgical referral is indicated. Unequal size of the scrotal contents may be because of hydrocele (transilluminates) (Figs 1.12, 1.13), larger varicocele, current or previous orchitis, or neoplasia. Longstanding varicoceles or small epididymal cysts (<1 cm) need not be investigated, but as ultrasound examination is cheap, easily available and without adverse effect, it is reasonable to have a fairly low threshold for investigation of any abnormality of the scrotal contents.

Rectum. Carry out perianal examination in all men with penile warts and all men who have sex with men. The patient lies in the left lateral position with the knees bent. Note the presence of warts (Fig. 1.14), excoriation, erythema or ulceration.

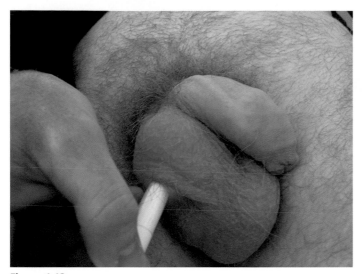

Figure 1.12
Transillumination of a scrotal hydrocele

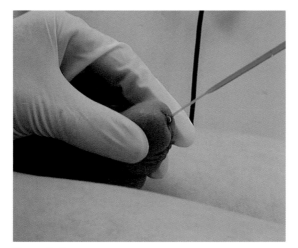

Figure 1.13
Plastic loop sample from the male urethra

Take microbiological samples for identification of *N. gonorrhoeae* and *C. trachomatis* from all men who have sex with men (MSM). 'Blind' samples can be taken from asymptomatic men (see Box 1.8). Perform proctoscopy in men with rectal symptoms. The proctoscope is lightly lubricated with jelly, pressed laterally for a few seconds at the anal margin and passed gently into the anal canal. Warts, ulceration or inflammation may be seen and microbiological samples can be taken under direct vision.

Urine. Do a dipstick test for the presence of blood, protein, glucose and nitrites at first attendance. A 'two-glass' urine test (Box 1.9) may be performed in men with:

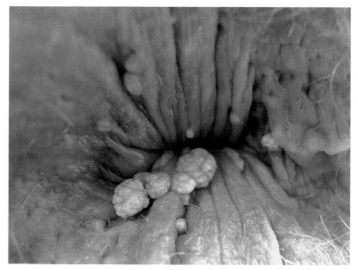

Figure 1.14
Perianal warts

Box 1.9: The 'two-glass' urine test

Visual examination of the urine for suspended pus cells (causing a cloudy urine that does not clear on the addition of 10% acetic acid), or casts of mucus or pus from the urethral glands suggests a diagnosis of urethritis. The 'two-glass' urine test, in which the presence of such casts in a first-voided urine sample, but absence in a second sample supports a diagnosis of anterior urethritis, may be useful where there are no facilities for microscopy or microbiological testing. The evidence base for the use of this test is poor, and its use in modern practice is in indicating that a patient should be referred for full examination and investigation of urethritis, rather than as a definitive diagnostic procedure.

- Symptoms of urethritis
- Contact of NSU/NSGI/PID/gonorrhoea (see Chs 2 and 4)
- Evidence of urethral discharge or inflammation
- Symptoms of prostatitis (see Ch. 5).

In men with symptoms of urinary-tract infection (UTI) and/or haematuria or proteinuria on dipstick testing, obtain a midstream urine sample for microscopy, culture and sensitivity. Ask the patient to wash his hands, retract the foreskin, pass a quantity of urine into the toilet (or provide an initial urine specimen for testing for *C. trachomatis*), then pass a sample into a sterile universal container.

Take blood samples from all men for syphilis serology and HIV testing (offer and discuss prior to testing – see Ch. 9). In men with risk factors for infection they are also required for hepatitis B and C serology and/or virology (see Ch. 8).

Specimen checklist: asymptomatic heterosexual man

- Urethral sample for Gram-stain microscopy
- Urethral sample for culture for *N. gonorrhoeae*
- Urethral sample or urine for testing for *C. trachomatis*
- Blood for syphilis screening serology
- Offer HIV antibody testing after discussion
- Check hepatitis B vaccination status, serology and vaccination if at risk.

Specimen checklist: asymptomatic homosexual man

- Oropharyngeal sample for culture for *N. gonorrhoeae*
- Urethral sample for Gram-stain microscopy
- Urethral sample for culture for *N. gonorrhoeae*
- Urethral sample or urine for testing for *C. trachomatis*
- Rectal sample for culture for *N. gonorrhoeae*
- Rectal sample for *C. trachomatis*
- Blood for syphilis screening serology
- Offer HIV antibody testing after discussion
- Check hepatitis A and B vaccination status, serology and vaccination.

ROUTINE EXAMINATION AND SPECIMEN COLLECTION IN WOMEN

Background

Women should be examined in the lithotomy position on a couch with stirrups or knee supports. Offer a gown or drape if possible, although many prefer to forgo these items.

Examination procedure

Take samples for the identification of *N. gonorrhoeae* from the pharynx (Box 1.10) in:

- Women who are contacts of gonorrhoea
- Women who have Gram-negative intracellular diplococci on urethral or cervical smear
- Sex workers.

Labia majora and minora. Gently separate the labia, noting the presence of skin lesions as above (Fig. 1.15), the presence and nature of any discharge and any erythema, oedema, lichenification or fissuring. Wipe away any discharge with a cotton wool ball.

Urethra and greater vestibular glands. Check for the presence of any urethral discharge. The openings of the greater vestibular glands, on the medial side of each labium minorum, may express secretions if the gland is massaged by a finger inserted into the vagina, palpating behind the labium majus. These can be smeared onto a glass slide for staining and microscopy. Microbiological specimens from the urethra for the identification of *N. gonorrhoeae* are required in all women (Fig. 1.16).

Tell the patient that you are about to pass the speculum before doing so. It should be lubricated with water and warmed to near body temperature if made of metal. Introduce

Box 1.10: Microbiological specimens in women

Pharynx

Use a cotton-tipped swab to sample material from both tonsils and tonsillar fossae, sweeping the swab quickly over the soft palate and uvula. Directly inoculate culture medium or place in charcoal medium for later plating for culture for *N. gonorrhoeae* (see Ch. 4).

Urethra

Use a plastic loop to sample material from the opening of the urethra. This can be quite painful, so warn the patient, take the sample slowly and without twisting the plastic loop. Smear a sample onto a glass slide for Gram staining and microscopy for identification of *N. gonorrhoeae* (either immediately, or air dried and sent with the patient to a clinic). Directly inoculate the culture medium using the same loop. If culture medium is unavailable, use a cotton-tipped swab and place in charcoal medium for later plating for culture for *N. gonorrhoeae*.

Vagina

Use a plastic loop or cotton-tipped swab to sample secretions from both lateral vaginal fornices and posterior fornix . Smear onto a glass microscope slide for Gram staining to classify the appearance of vaginal bacteria, identify spores of *Candida* species and hyphae. Take a second sample and mix with a drop of saline on a second microscope slide for microscopy for identification of clue cells and *T. vaginalis* (see Ch. 3).

Additional samples may be taken from the same sites and placed in Amies transport medium or directly onto culture plates for culture for *Candida* spp. or *T. vaginalis* (see Ch. 3).

Cervix

a) Use a cotton wool mop held in sponge forceps to remove excess secretions from the endocervix.
b) Use a plastic loop or cotton-tipped swab to sample material from the endocervical canal. Smear a sample onto a glass slide for Gram staining and microscopy, then smear directly onto a culture plate for *N. gonorrhoeae*. If culture medium unavailable place in charcoal medium for later plating for culture for *N. gonorrhoeae*.
c) Use a cotton-tipped swab, rotated in the endocervix for 15 s, to obtain material for testing for *C. trachomatis*.

Rectum

Use a cotton wool swab (dry, or moistened with sterile saline) passed about 3 cm into the anal canal to obtain a sample from the anal canal and the terminal rectum for culture for *N. gonorrhoeae*.

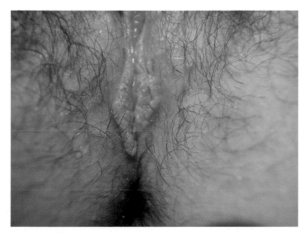

Figure 1.15
Warts on the female perineum

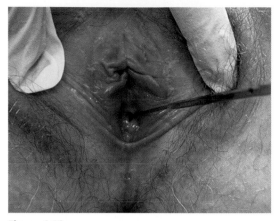

Figure 1.16
Plastic loop sample from the female urethra

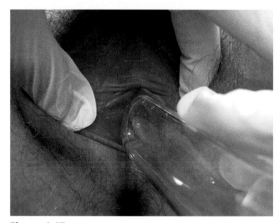

Figure 1.17
Introducing the speculum in the vertical plane

the speculum slowly (Fig. 1.17), parting the labia with one hand, pressing gently against the hymenal remnants with the fully closed blades in the near vertical plane, avoiding catching pubic hairs or pressing on the mons. Rotate the speculum into the horizontal position as it is inserted. Check that the patient is not in discomfort, then warn the patient before opening the speculum gently to reveal the cervix. If the cervix is not immediately visible, don't open the blades any wider. Asking the patient to cough, tilting the pelvis forward by asking the patient to place her hands under her lower back, or withdrawing and re-inserting the speculum may help. If unsuccessful, withdraw the speculum and locate the cervix by bimanual examination before inserting the speculum again.

Vagina. Look for warts or erythema of the vaginal mucosa. Note the nature, colour and smell of discharge (Fig. 1.18).

Microbiological specimens from the vagina are required in all women (Box 1.10).

Cervix. Assess normal cervical anatomy: size, os, presence or absence of cervical ectropion, Nabothian cysts, cervical mucus or intrauterine contraceptive device (IUCD)

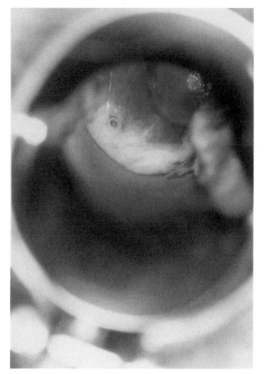

Figure 1.18
Physiological vaginal discharge

threads. Note cervical abnormalities: presence of warts or ulceration, scarring or evidence of previous laser or diathermy, mucopurulent or purulent cervical discharge, cervical inflammation, bleeding.

Microbiological specimens from the cervix are required in all women (Box 1.10).

Perineum and perianal area. Look for ulceration, excoriation, warts.

Bimanual vaginal examination. This may not be necessary in all women, but perform in all symptomatic women, asymptomatic women with an STI diagnosis and women who are contacts of men with STI. Insert the lubricated gloved index and middle fingers of one hand into the vagina, locating the cervix. Palpate the abdomen with the other hand. Cervical motion tenderness (also termed cervical excitation) is (quite severe) pain on movement of the cervix. Tenderness and/or masses in the adnexae can be detected by simultaneously palpating the lateral vaginal fornices with the examining hand while the other hand presses deep in the iliac fossae.

Rectum. Microbiological specimens are required from the rectum in all women (Box 1.10).

Urine is required:

- In women who are concerned about pregnancy, or where the differential diagnosis includes intrauterine or ectopic pregnancy. Test a sample of urine (preferably early morning) with a commercial test kit. Most kits will detect pregnancy within 10 days of a missed period

- In women with symptoms of urinary tract infection (UTI) and/or haematuria or proteinuria on multistix testing. Take a midstream urine sample for microscopy, culture and sensitivity. Ask the patient to wash her hands, hold the labia apart, pass a quantity of urine into the toilet (or provide an initial urine specimen for testing for *C. trachomatis*), then pass a sample into a sterile universal container.

Take blood samples from all women for syphilis serology and HIV testing (offer and discuss prior to testing – see Ch. 9). In women with risk factors for infection they are also required for hepatitis B and C serology and/or virology (Ch. 8).

Specimen checklist: asymptomatic women

- Urethral sample for culture for *N. gonorrhoeae*
- Endocervical sample or urine for testing for *C. trachomatis*
- Endocervical sample for culture for *N. gonorrhoeae*
- Wet mount vaginal slide for *T. vaginalis*
- Rectal sample for culture for *N. gonorrhoeae*
- Blood for syphilis screening serology
- Offer HIV antibody testing after discussion
- Check hepatitis B vaccination status, serology and vaccination if at risk.

Further Reading

Burtney E. Teenage sexuality in Scotland. Edinburgh; Health Education Board for Scotland: 2000 (available at www.hebs.scot.nhs.uk/research).

Confidentiality and people under 16, BMA, Brook, FPA, GMSC, HEA and RCGP Joint Guidance, 1993.

Graney DO, Lontver LA. Anatomy and physical examination of the female genital tract. In: Holmes KK, Starling PF et al (eds). Sexually transmitted diseases, 3rd edn. New York; McGraw-Hill; 1999: pp. 685–698.

Johnson AM, Mercer CH, Erens B et al. Sexual behaviour in Britain: partnerships, practices and risk behaviour. Lancet 2001; 358: 1835–1842.

Kreiger JN, Graney DO. Clinical anatomy, histology and physical examination of the male genital tract. In: Holmes KK, Starling PF et al (eds). Sexually transmitted diseases, 3rd edn. New York; McGraw-Hill; 1999: pp. 699–710.

Neighbour R. The inner consultation. Edinburgh; Churchill Livingstone: 1987.

PHLS, DHSS & PS and the Scottish ISD (D)5 Collaborative Group. Sexually transmitted infections in the UK: New episodes seen at genitourinary medicine clinics, 1991–2001. London; Public Health Laboratory Service: 2002.

Pryce A. 'Does your mother know you are heterosexual?': discretion management and resistance of the erotic in the genitourinary clinic. Crit Pub Health 2000; 10: 295-311.

Tate P. The doctor's communication handbook. Oxford; Radcliffe Medical Press: 1997.

Wellings K, Field J, Johnson AM, Wadsworth J. Sexual behaviour in Britain: the national survey of sexual attitudes and lifestyle. London; Penguin Books: 1994.

SELF-ASSESSMENT

Louise (13 years) attends the clinic asking for a test for *Chlamydia*. She is reluctant to discuss why she wants a test.

Questions

a) Note down some of the things you might try to explore at the beginning of the consultation.

She later discloses that she has a regular boyfriend who is 17 years old. They have been together for 6 weeks. She has had three previous partners aged between 16 and 20. Last week she had sex with her partner's friend who is 18 years old.

b) What else do you need to know?
c) What are the priorities? What else might you wish to discuss with her?

Answers

a) Explore the reason for her concern and understanding of chlamydial infection. Why is she concerned just now? How did she find out about the clinic? Has someone come with her? General questions about what she already knows about the clinic or how she found it may open up a narrative that can be directed towards her underlying concern. You may wish to discuss confidentiality at this point. It may also be sensible to state the limits of confidentiality if you feel that there is a child protection issue – although this may inhibit her from disclosing details. If possible discuss the presence of and details of symptoms. Direct questions about discharge, pain, post-coital and intermenstrual bleeding may be required. Ask about current and previous partners (age of partners and nature of relationship). Find out about her use and knowledge of contraception and protection. What are her social circumstances (home situation, support, self-esteem, mood)? Does she have a close relative, guardian, friend or group of friends or other support network?

b) When did she last have sex? Under what circumstances does sex usually take place? Find out about her use of alcohol and other recreational drugs. Although sex is likely to have been consensual, explore whether there is evidence of coercion, force or payment. Does her partner know about her having sex with his friend and under what circumstances did this arise? What are her feelings about pregnancy?

c) Your priorities might be to:
   - clarify and address the patient's agenda
   - decide if there is a child protection issue (seek advice from senior colleagues if necessary)
   - discuss the extent and limits of confidentiality
   - do a pregnancy test
   - address immediate contraceptive needs
   - involve a health adviser or other colleague
   - offer examination and explain it in detail. A urine test for chlamydial infection is a non-invasive alternative
   - suggest she confides in a parent or carer (see Gillick competence)
   - refer to other agencies (e.g. social work) or sources of support
   - try to arrange follow-up.

Non-gonococcal urethritis, chlamydial infection and pelvic inflammatory disease

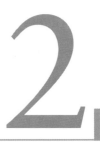

INTRODUCTION

Urethral discharge is one of the commonest problems seen in men in genitourinary medical practice. In most clinics in the UK and the USA, the majority of these men will have non-gonococcal urethritis (NGU). In women, the most important complication of an STI is pelvic inflammatory disease (PID). The aetiology of these and related conditions, including mucopurulent cervicitis in women and epididymo-orchitis in men, is thought to be similar but is incompletely understood. *Chlamydia trachomatis* is the organism most commonly isolated in clinical practice, although these clinical syndromes are multifactorial (Box 2.1). *C. trachomatis* also infects the rectum causing proctitis in men and women; ocular infection causes non-gonococcal ophthalmia neonatorum in newborns and conjunctivitis in adults. PID and its sequelae, which include chronic pain, ectopic pregnancy and tubal infertility, have enormous social and financial impacts. The most important causes worldwide are *N. gonorrhoeae* and *C. trachomatis* infections, although in parts of the world such as the UK, where gonorrhoea is much less common, chlamydial infection is responsible for up to 50% of acute cases. Most significantly, *C. trachomatis* is asymptomatic in 50% of men and in up to 80% of women, in whom it is estimated to be responsible for one-third of all cases of tubal infertility and the majority of cases of ectopic pregnancy. Most women with these complications have no history of symptomatic PID. Public awareness of *Chlamydia* and its sequelae is increasing rapidly and greater numbers of asymptomatic individuals request information on and testing for *C. trachomatis*. Alternatives to testing and treatment in GU clinics, including postal testing kits (see Figs 2.1, 2.2) and mass-screening programmes, are being explored in the UK.

TERMINOLOGY

Non-gonococcal urethritis (NGU) in men is also termed non-specific urethritis (NSU). In true non-specific urethritis, no cause can be found, so NGU is the better term. Men with NGU may have symptoms of urethritis or may be asymptomatic; microscopy of Gram-stained specimens of their urethral discharge reveals pus cells but no Gram-negative intracellular diplococci. *C. trachomatis* is detected in 20–50% of men with NGU, although there is good evidence that *Ureaplasma urealyticum*, *Mycoplasma genitalium* and perhaps

Box 2.1: Clinical syndromes associated with Chlamydia trachomatis

Clinical presentation	Causative organism(s)
Non-gonococcal urethritis (NGU)/ non-specific urethritis (NSU)/ non-specific genital infection (NSGI) (male)	Experimental evidence: *C. trachomatis* *Ureaplasma urealyticum* *Mycoplasma genitalium*
	Clinical experience suggests: Herpes simplex virus *Trichomonas vaginalis* *Candida* spp. Coliforms associated with urinary tract infection
	Possible: *Mycoplasma hominis* *Haemophilus influenzae* Organisms associated with bacterial vaginosis Non-infective causes
Post-gonococcal urethritis	*C. trachomatis* ? *U. urealyticum* ? *M. genitalium*
NSGI (women)	*C. trachomatis* ? *U. urealyticum* ? *M. genitalium*
Pelvic inflammatory disease	*C. trachomatis* (*N. gonorrhoeae*) (see Ch. 4) Organisms associated with bacterial vaginosis ? *M. hominis* ? *M. genitalium* ? *U. urealyticum*
Ophthalmia neonatorum	*C. trachomatis* (*N. gonorrhoeae*) ? *M. hominis* ? organisms associated with bacterial vaginosis
Epididymitis (Ch. 5)	*C. trachomatis* (*N. gonorrhoeae*) Enteric organisms
Reactive arthritis (Ch. 5) Adult conjunctivitis	*C. trachomatis*

other organisms are involved. *C. trachomatis* can also infect the urethra, endocervix and Bartholin's glands in women, but the symptoms and signs of lower genital-tract infection in women are less clearly correlated with infective aetiology. Non-specific genital infection (NSGI) is an unsatisfactory term intended to include lower genital-tract infections in both sexes.

PATHOGENESIS AND CLINICAL PRACTICE

Chlamydiae have previously been classified as protozoans and later as viruses, but are now recognized as bacteria. They are obligate intracellular parasites, depending on the

29

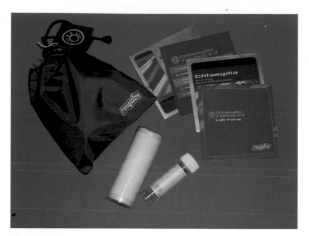

Figure 2.1
Postal testing kit for *Chlamydia* and contents: urine container, protective sleeve, envelope for postage to laboratory and instructions

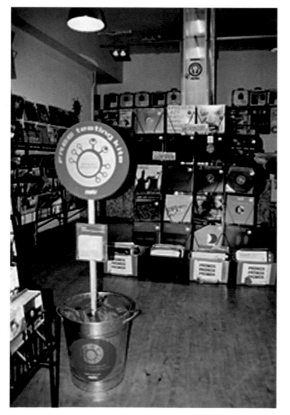

Figure 2.2
Pick-up point for *Chlamydia* postal testing kits in a record store

host cell to supply energy as ATP. Samples for tests for chlamydial infection should, therefore, contain cellular material.

U. urealyticum is isolated in 20% to 80% of men with NGU in clinical studies, but also from similar numbers of men without NGU who are matched for sexual activity. Studies with antibiotics active against *U. urealyticum,* but not against *C. trachomatis* and vice-versa suggest that *U. urealyticum* does have a role in the pathogenesis of NGU. For example, rifampicin and sulphonamides are active against *C. trachomatis* but not *U. urealyticum.* Men with symptomatic NGU in whom *U. urealyticum* is isolated but *C. trachomatis* is not, respond poorly to treatment with these antibiotics. *M. genitalium* is also found more frequently in urethral samples of men with urethritis than those without, and causes urethritis in chimpanzees, however, evidence for a causal role in man is lacking. It has been suggested that the organisms causing bacterial vaginosis in women are also responsible for some cases of NGU, but this is unproven.

There is evidence that many people spontaneously clear chlamydial infection and that some immunity to re-infection develops. Those who do not clear an initial infection, or fail to develop immunity and acquire repeat infections are at risk of sequelae. *C. trachomatis* is a powerful immunogen and those with current or past infection develop a cellular immune response. This response is enhanced in those clearing chlamydial infection spontaneously, but appears to be depressed in those who develop complications. It has been postulated that an autoimmune mechanism is involved in *Chlamydia*-induced damage to both the eye and the genital tract. Antibodies to a 60kDa chlamydial heat-shock protein (HSP60) are found in 50% of women with PID and cross-react with human heat-shock protein (HSP60). In women with chlamydial PID, presence of HSP60 antibodies is associated with a past history of PID, proven tubal occlusion, presence of adhesions and a degree of tubal inflammation at laparoscopy. It is not clear whether these antibodies are responsible for the chronic immune system stimulation implicated in *Chlamydia*-induced damage, or whether they merely reflect chronic persistent infection. *C. trachomatis* infection persisting for at least a year has been observed in infants. Recent evidence using gene sequencing of isolates from women repeatedly diagnosed with chlamydial infection over several years suggests that persistent infection may also occur in the human genital tract.

NON-GONOCOCCAL URETHRITIS/NON-SPECIFIC URETHRITIS

The distinction between gonococcal and non-gonococcal urethritis became possible with the identification and culture of *N. gonorrhoeae* in the 1880s onwards, although cell culture for isolation of *C. trachomatis* was not available until 1965. Approximately 10% of men attending genitourinary medicine clinics in the UK are diagnosed with non-gonococcal urethritis (NGU). The aetiology of NGU is summarized in Box 2.2.

CLINICAL FEATURES

Follow the procedure for routine history taking and examination in Chapter 1.

Box 2.2: Aetiology of NGU

Organism	Isolated in (% of cases)	Estimated causal in (% of cases)
Chlamydia trachomatis	20–50%	20–50%
Ureaplasma urealyticum	20–80%	10–20%
Mycoplasma genitalium	10–30%	10–20%
Trichomonas vaginalis	1–17%	[1]
Other organisms: Herpes simplex *Candida* spp. Coliforms associated with UTI	Rare	Rare
Non-infective: Trauma/foreign body Other causes[2]		Rare
No cause found: 'true' non-specific urethritis	20–50%	20–50%

[1]The proportion of cases attributable to *Trichomonas vaginalis* is related to prevalence in the community and is low in most parts of the UK.
[2]Other causes including alcohol, allergy, abstinence, excess sexual activity, dehydration and masturbation have been blamed.

Symptoms

- NGU may be asymptomatic
- When present, symptoms are those of urethritis, occurring 1–5 weeks after sexual contact
- A clear, creamy white, yellow or green discharge occurs with or without dysuria. Urethral itch or discomfort may be the only symptom
- The incubation period of NGU is often longer, and the discharge less purulent, than that of gonococcal urethritis, but these differences do not permit diagnosis on clinical grounds
- Occasionally men presenting with NGU will give no history of sexual contact
- Be aware of the occasional co-existence of conjunctival infection, reactive arthritis or epididymo-orchitis in men with NGU.

Clinical notes: history taking in urethral discharge

- Symptoms: discharge, dysuria, testicular pain
- Last sexual contact: casual/regular, gender, location
- Other sexual contacts
- Drug history and allergies.

Examination

The best time for examination is first thing in the morning, after holding the urine overnight. Convention is that examination for suspected urethritis should take place at least 4 hours after last passing urine, but the optimal time is unknown.

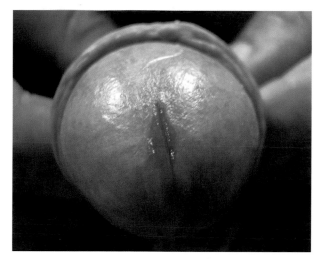

Figure 2.3
Inflammation of the urethral meatus in NGU

Discharge may be visible at the meatus or on the underwear (Fig. 2.3).

Examine the testes and epididymi carefully for evidence of epididymo-orchitis.

In men who have symptoms suggesting urethritis but no evidence of urethritis on examination and microscopy, recall for a repeat examination in the morning, having held urine overnight. This procedure is known as the 'early morning smear' (EMS).

INVESTIGATIONS

A sample of discharge expressed from the urethra, or from a 10 μl plastic loop swab inserted 2–3 cm into the urethra should be smeared onto a microscope slide, covering about 1 cm^2.

Tests on urethral or first-voided urine samples are mandatory for the identification of *C. trachomatis* and *N. gonorrhoeae*.

Test a midstream sample of urine with a dipstick that detects protein, blood, glucose, nitrites and leukocyte esterase. In some clinics this test is restricted to men with symptoms suggesting possible UTI. Samples positive for the last two tests should be sent for microscopy and culture.

Facilities for identifying *U. urealyticum* and *M. genitalis* are not usually routinely available.

The 'two-glass' urine test, consisting of first-passed urine (FPU) and midstream urine has been used for diagnosing urethritis. Threads (casts of mucus or mucopus washed from the urethral glands) in the first sample but none in the midstream is supportive of urethritis. The test's main use in modern practice is to obtain threads for Gram staining and microscopy.

Microscopy

Any of the following findings give a presumptive diagnosis of NGU, although definitive diagnosis requires the exclusion of gonococcal urethritis by negative culture for gonococcus.

Gram stain the urethral smear and examine first under low power to find areas with the most polymorphonuclear leucocytes (PMNL). At $1000 \times$ magnification with the oil immersion lens, the presence of five or more PMNLs (pus cells) in at least five high power fields in the absence of Gram-negative intracellular diplococci gives a diagnosis of NGU.

If the patient has symptoms suggestive of NGU and a negative slide, the presence of more than five pus cells, as described above, in a specimen obtained after holding urine overnight ('early morning smear') gives a presumptive diagnosis of NGU.

A urethral 'thread' is taken from a first-passed urine (FPU) sample using a plastic loop. This is prepared and Gram stained in the same way as a urethral smear. The presence of ten or more PMNLs per high power field is diagnostic of NGU.

A first-passed urine specimen is centrifuged at 400 g for 10 minutes and resuspended in 0.5 ml of urine. This is plated out and Gram stained in the same way as a urethral smear. The presence of more than ten PMNLs per high power field is diagnostic of NGU.

Rarer causes of urethritis are given in Box 2.3.

Box 2.3: Rarer causes of urethritis

Herpes simplex virus (HSV) urethritis

When urethral discharge is accompanied by flu-like systemic symptoms or groin, buttock or leg pain, consider the possibility of HSV urethritis. Severe dysuria with scant discharge can also point to this diagnosis. Where routine testing for HSV antigen has taken place, herpes is found in up to 10% of cases of NGU and may be an under-recognized cause of the condition. Other features include:

- Severe dysuria
- Bloodstained discharge (sometimes with haematuria)
- Inguinal lymphadenopathy
- Intrameatal ulceration.

The clinical picture may be difficult to distinguish from urinary-tract infection. If the diagnosis is suspected, take a plastic loop urethral specimen in viral transport medium for HSV isolation. After obtaining routine samples for other STIs it is reasonable to treat on clinical suspicion with short course aciclovir/famciclovir/valaciclovir (Ch. 6).

Urethritis associated with urinary tract infection

When discharge is accompanied by frequency, haematuria, abdominal pain, severe dysuria and/or systemic symptoms, consider urethritis associated with UTI. Microscopy of a Gram-stained, mid-stream clean-catch urine with more than one bacterium per high-power field supports the diagnosis.

- Confirm that Gram-stained slide of urethral smear contains pus cells but no Gram-negative diplococci (GNDC)
- Use a dipstick to test for haematuria, proteinuria and presence of nitrites and leukocyte esterase in a midstream urine sample
- Send a sterile midstream sample of urine for culture and sensitivity
- Do standard tests to exclude sexually transmitted infection
- Treat for UTI with single-dose or short-course antibiotic therapy.

All male patients with proven UTI should have renal-tract imaging or be referred for urological investigation to exclude structural abnormality of the urological tract.

Simon (19 years) complained of a week's history of green urethral discharge. He had passed urine 30 minutes before being examined in the clinic. A Gram-stained urethral smear contained 3–5 PMNLs per high power field. He was re-examined the following morning when the slide contained more than twenty PMNLs per field, but no Gram-negative intracellular diplococci (GNID). He was treated with azithromycin 1 g single dose and his three sexual partners in the previous month were traced.

Treatment

Treat as for uncomplicated chlamydial infection (see Box 2.7). The cure rate of single dose azithromycin 1 g or of a week's course of doxycycline 100 mg twice daily is comparable in chlamydial and in non-chlamydial NGU (level of evidence 1b). The cure rate of *U. urealyticum* associated NGU is lower with either regimen than when *C. trachomatis* is isolated. Some experts recommend that a week or more of antibiotic therapy reduces the likelihood of recurrent or persistent NGU, but the evidence for this is lacking.

COUNSELLING, INFORMATION AND PARTNER NOTIFICATION

Information

Give information on NGU, chlamydial infection and its implications. Reinforce advice with written information in the form of a leaflet.

- The importance of treatment of female partner(s), regardless of test results should be stressed
- There is no known effect on male fertility. However, men are sometimes concerned regarding the effect on the fertility of a current or past female partner and this should be discussed
- Arrange for follow-up 2–3 weeks after completion of therapy.

PARTNER NOTIFICATION

Where available, all men with NGU should be referred to a trained health adviser (HA) on diagnosis. They should be offered a choice of self-notification, provider notification or conditional notification.

Treatment of contacts of men with NGU

Symptomatic men. All partners within the last month should be seen and offered treatment – because men who develop symptoms of NGU usually do so within a month of acquiring infection.

Asymptomatic men. All partners within the last 6 months, or the most recent partner, should be seen and offered treatment. (This may be interpreted according to microbiological findings. Greater priority should be given to tracing female contacts of men with *Chlamydia*-positive NGU.)

Female partners of men with NGU should be treated whether or not *Chlamydia* is isolated (evidence level 1b).

Standard advice is to avoid intercourse until follow-up appointment. If a man with NGU and his only partner are treated simultaneously, there is no reason why intercourse should not resume once symptoms have resolved.

Follow-up

- Men with NGU should be reviewed 2–3 weeks after treatment to confirm resolution of symptoms and treatment of sexual contacts
- Results of tests for other infections will be available at this time
- Routine repeat microscopy of the urethral smear is not indicated in men whose symptoms have resolved.

RECURRENT AND PERSISTENT NGU

Recurrent or persistent NGU is reported to follow in 1–60% of acute cases. Diagnosis is based on a microscopic diagnosis of NGU according to the standard criteria, in the presence or absence of symptoms, at least 10 days after treatment. In asymptomatic men, other than those with HIV serodiscordant partners, there is no proven advantage to either patient or female partner in retreating recurrent or persistent NGU. Repeat investigation and intervention is often unsuccessful, likely to increase anxiety, and should probably be confined to clinical research. Reserve investigation for men with recurrent or persisting symptoms. Some men presenting with persistent or recurrent symptoms of NGU will have objective evidence of continuing or recurrent urethral inflammation, but many will not. An outline of the management of these men with persisting or recurrent symptoms is given in Figure 2.4. There is currently insufficient evidence on which to form a consensus on management of recurrent and persistent NGU, so there are wide variations in clinical practice. A detailed history, rather than immediate examination and repeat microscopy in a rushed clinic, may give pointers to the likelihood for the need for repeat treatment. Time spent on a first return consultation can help to minimize problems in the future, in identifying those men who have symptoms of a functional origin, often related to anxieties about their own or a partner's suspected infidelity. If symptomatic men are to be re-examined to exclude persistent or recurrent NGU, an early morning smear allows a definitive decision on whether inflammation persists.

Case history

Steven (27 years) presented with a discharge in the mornings, 4 weeks after epidemiological treatment for chlamydial infection discovered when his regular partner was tested at a routine smear appointment. The nurse at the GUM clinic established that he had researched extensively on the internet and was squeezing his penis daily to check whether discharge was present. A Gram-stained urethral smear showed epithelial cells only and he was reassured – and dissuaded from squeezing.

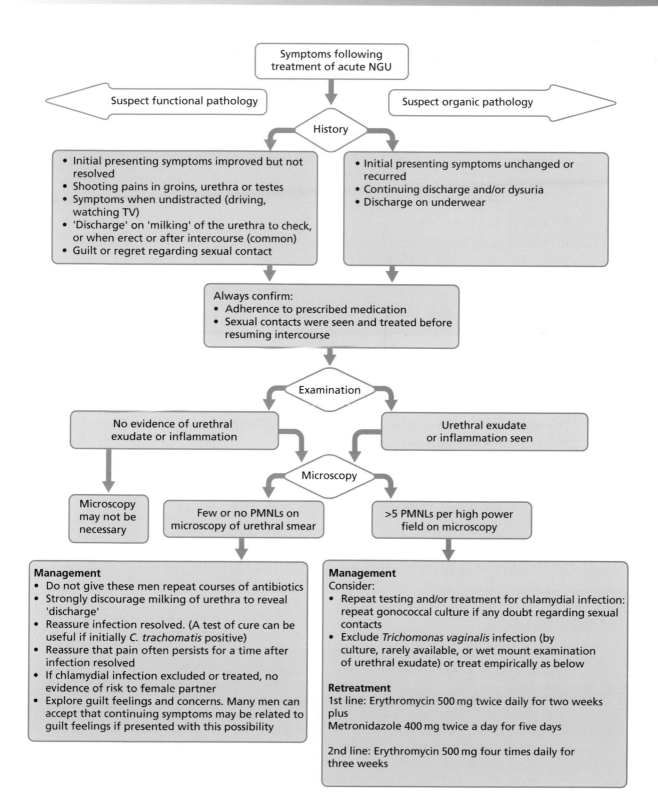

Figure 2.4
Management of recurrent NGU

PATHOGENESIS AND CLINICAL PRACTICE

Chemotactic markers of inflammation persist for weeks after treatment of acute NGU and are less marked in chlamydial than in non-chlamydial NGU.

The type of antibiotic used and the duration of treatment in the management of acute NGU does not affect the probability of development of recurrent or persistent NGU.

Reinfection with, and persistence of, *C. trachomatis* appears to be rare, but both *M. genitalium* and *U. urealyticum* have been implicated as causing persistent or recurrent NGU. A persistent immune response to chlamydial heat-shock protein HSP60 has also been suggested as a cause.

Persistent NGU, whether symptomatic or asymptomatic, does not cause structural damage to the urethra or affect fertility.

POST-GONOCOCCAL URETHRITIS

Men treated for gonorrhoea with penicillin, ciprofloxacin or aminoglycosides may have a recurrence of discharge containing polymorphonuclear leukocytes (PMNLs) but no *N. gonorrhoeae* on microscopy or culture. This may reflect the longer incubation period of infection with *C. trachomatis* compared to that of *N. gonorrhoeae* . The aetiology of this condition appears to be similar to that of NGU, although the role of *U. urealyticum* and other *Mycoplasma* spp. is even less clear.

Approximately 25% of heterosexual men with urethral *N. gonorrhoeae* infection are co-infected with *C. trachomatis* and it is common practice to give treatment for both organisms when *N. gonorrhoeae* is identified. Co-infection is less common in homosexual men in most settings.

NON-SPECIFIC GENITAL INFECTION IN WOMEN

BACKGROUND

In women, the association between symptoms and signs of urogenital infection and infective aetiology is not clearly defined. The presence of multiple pathogens or potential pathogens in symptomatic women is common. The diagnostic label non-specific genital infection (NSGI) is attached to two distinct groups of women:

1. *Symptomatic women and those with clinical signs.* In women with vaginal discharge, pain or dysuria, and in some asymptomatic women, there may be clinical evidence of mucopurulent cervicitis, urethritis, or rarely vaginitis or Bartholinitis, attributable to suspected infection with organisms implicated in NGU in men. They are treated with antibiotics active against *C. trachomatis*, but may also require treatment with antibiotics active against facultative bacteria and anaerobes associated with bacterial vaginosis.

2. *Asymptomatic women without clinical signs.* Women with no symptoms or signs of infection but who are contacts of men with NGU, are treated with antibiotics active against *C. trachomatis* and other organisms implicated in NGU; this is done for two reasons:

- because about 60% of women who are contacts of men with chlamydial NGU, and over 20% of women who are contacts of non-chlamydial NGU, will be infected with *C. trachomatis*
- because such women are assumed to be asymptomatic carriers of organisms implicated in NGU in men.

The implications of carriage of *U. urealyticum* and *M. genitalium* in women, other than the risk of reinfecting a male partner, are not understood. We do not yet know whether these organisms are responsible for some of the 50% of cases of pelvic inflammatory disease in which neither *N. gonorrhoeae* nor *C. trachomatis* is isolated.

CLINICAL FEATURES

A full history, examination and testing for sexually transmitted infections is indicated as outlined in Chapter 1.

Symptoms

Women may present as asymptomatic contacts of men with NGU or with vaginal discharge (Ch. 3), dysuria or pain.

Signs

A mucopurulent (yellow) discharge (Fig. 2.5) on an endocervical swab, or increased numbers of polymorphs on microscopy of endocervical mucus has been associated with an increased probability of chlamydial or gonococcal infection in several studies. These findings, together with cervical bleeding on taking endocervical specimens, are sometimes taken as evidence for empirical treatment for *C. trachomatis* in asymptomatic women at risk of infection. However, clinical diagnosis, even by those with extensive clinical experience is no substitute for microbiological testing.

Do a bimanual examination in symptomatic women to check for signs of pelvic inflammatory disease.

TREATMENT

Asymptomatic contacts of men with NGU with no adnexal tenderness or cervical motion tenderness on bimanual examination should be treated for chlamydial infection only.

Women with pelvic pain or symptoms suggestive of pelvic inflammatory disease and adnexal tenderness or cervical motion tenderness on bimanual examination should be treated for pelvic inflammatory disease (see Box 2.11, p. 49).

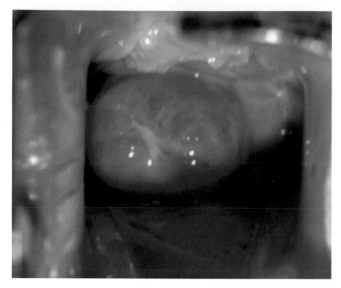

Figure 2.5
Mucopurulent cervicitis

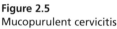

Case history

Michelle, aged 16, reluctantly presented with a change in vaginal discharge and some post-coital bleeding of three weeks' duration. Examination revealed an inflamed cervix that bled when touched and a mucopurulent cervical discharge, but no pelvic tenderness. Gram-stain microscopy of endocervical, urethral and vaginal swabs showed no evidence of GNID or bacterial vaginosis; wet mount microscopy revealed no trichomoniasis. She was treated for possible chlamydial infection with azithromycin 1 g single dose.

Comment: Although the ideal is to treat only microbiologically proven infection, a pragmatic approach is sometimes appropriate, based on knowledge of the prevalence of infections in at-risk groups and the likelihood of attendance for follow-up.

PATIENT INFORMATION

The information given to women should depend on the microbiological findings. Written information covering both NGU and chlamydial infection is useful for women counselled before microbiological results are available, or where patient confidentiality prevents disclosure of microbiological findings in the male. The following points may need discussion:

- There is no evidence of any effect on fertility in women who are contacts of non-chlamydial NGU
- Treatment may have reduced the chance of developing PID, although this is not proven
- The development of NGU in a male partner is not evidence of infidelity in a regular relationship
- Women in whom *C. trachomatis* is isolated, or who are contacts of men with chlamydial NGU, should be advised as for chlamydial infection.

CHLAMYDIAL INFECTION

BACKGROUND

Chlamydia trachomatis is one of four species of the genus *Chlamydia*, three of which are human pathogens. The acceptable abbreviation '*Chlamydia*' is often used in sexual health circles and, with greater awareness of sexual health in the media, increasingly in everyday language. It usually refers to a sexually transmitted infection with genital serovars of *C. trachomatis*. *C. trachomatis* is the commonest bacterial STI worldwide with 89 million cases per annum. In most populations the prevalence is highest in teenage women and in men in their early 20s (Box 2.4). Prevalence reduces with age in both sexes, probably partly due to the development of immunity. *Chlamydia* is a relatively uncommon finding in women over the age of 35. There is much less evidence relating to chlamydial prevalence in men. Reported rates in men are almost always lower than those in women of the same age.

Transmission

C. trachomatis can infect a number of sites in humans (Box 2.5).

Hyperendemic trachoma, caused by biovar trachoma, is transmitted from eye to eye. The lymphogranuloma venereum (LGV) biovar of *Chlamydia* is always sexually transmitted (Ch. 9). Non-endemic trachoma serovars, which are the cause of most oculogenital infections, are usually sexually transmitted. Repeated sexual contact with an infected partner carries a 70% chance of transmission, but the risk of transmission from a single exposure is unknown. Genital discharges in adults may be transferred during sex or by hand contamination to the eye, causing chlamydial conjunctivitis (Fig. 2.6). Newborn babies may develop chlamydial conjunctivitis or chlamydial pneumonia as a result of vertical transmission during passage through an infected birth canal.

Box 2.4: *Prevalence of chlamydial infection*

Population sampled	Prevalence
Sexually active women, UK	
National population sample, 15–44 years	1.5%
Attending general practice for any reason,	
all women	3–5%
women under 25	8%
women under 20	10%
Attending termination, antenatal or gynaecology outpatient clinics	5%
Attending GUM clinics	7–30%
Sexually active men, UK	
National population sample, 15–44 years	2.2%
Heterosexual men attending GUM clinics	9–15%
Unselected military recruits	11%
Homosexual men attending GUM clinics (urethral)	2%
(rectal)	5–10%

Box 2.5: Sites of C. trachomatis *infection*

Site	Prevalence and symptoms
Male urethra	Found in 2–15% of male GU clinic attendees Asymptomatic in 50% Cause of 20–50% of NGU in heterosexual men
Female urethra	Accompanies cervical infection in up to 75% of women but rarely symptomatic. May be a cause of 'sterile' pyuria
Endocervix	In 5–10% of sexually active women under 25 in most settings Up to 80% of urogenital infections are asymptomatic Of women with urogenital *Chlamydia* infection, 90% have infection of the cervix
Rectum (male and female)	Chlamydiae infect the rectum in approximately 5% of women and 5–10% of homosexual men attending GUM clinics Symptoms occur in less than half of the cases, and include anal discharge, bleeding and perianal pain
Pharynx (male and female)	Appears to be rare (<2%) and usually asymptomatic in both women and homosexual men
Conjunctiva (adults)	Usually a unilateral conjunctivitis. Caused by direct or manual transfer of genital *Chlamydia* infection (which often co-exists) to the eye
Conjunctiva (neonates)	See Appendix

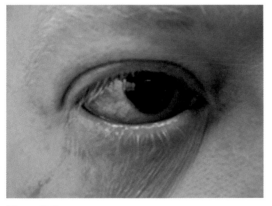

Figure 2.6
Chlamydial conjunctivitis

Methods of detecting Chlamydia

Until the mid 1990s the accepted gold standard test for *C. trachomatis* was culture, either in the egg yolk-sac or an immortal cell culture line. Although specificity of this test was very high, the sensitivity is now known to be relatively low. Nucleic acid amplification tests (NAAT) are more sensitive, and more specific than previously available tests and are now widely available. However, newly developed antigen detection methods have cost advantages and may approach the sensitivity of DNA methods. Methods of combining different tests – for example, using enzyme immunoassay (EIA) as a screening test with a confirmatory NAAT performed on samples with equivocal results – or pooling samples for NAAT testing to reduce costs, are also being explored.

Methods for detecting *C. trachomatis* are compared in Box 2.6.

Treatment

First-line treatment for uncomplicated chlamydial infection is with doxycycline or azithromycin (Box 2.7). Meta-analyses of clinical trials suggest that these drugs have

Box 2.6: Advantages and disadvantages of detection methods for C. trachomatis

Method	Advantages	Disadvantages
Nucleic acid based tests	High sensitivity (90–100%) and specificity (99%) Non-invasive specimens – urine or self-taken vulval swabs Novel testing strategies (e.g. by post)	Cost Inhibitors may affect results (urine tests in pregnancy) Contamination risk
Culture methods	High specificity Legally recognized	Low sensitivity Dependent upon quality of specimen collection, transport and culture technique and expertise of operator
Direct fluorescent antibody	High specificity Useful as confirmatory test	Operator dependent Lower sensitivity in male urethral samples
Enzyme immunoassay	Near patient testing (solid phase) Rapid result Inexpensive Can be used on male urine samples Simple Results objective Automatable	Low sensitivity of some tests Not suitable for female urine samples

Box 2.7: Treatment of uncomplicated chlamydial infection

1st line	Azithromycin 1 g single dose (1a) or doxycycline 100 mg twice daily for 7 days (1a)
2nd line	Ofloxacin 200 mg or 300 mg twice daily for 7 days (1b) or ofloxacin 400 mg once daily for 7 days (1b) or minocycline 100 mg once daily for 9 days
3rd line	Erythromycin 500 mg twice daily for 7 days (1b) or erythromycin 500 mg four times daily for 7 days (1b) or oxytetracycline 250 mg four times daily for 7 days (1b)

(Data from Horner and Owen Caul, 2002; Centers for Disease Control and Prevention, 2002 and SIGN, 2000.)

equal efficacy. A number of other tetracycline, macrolide and quinolone antibiotics are known to be over 95% effective in achieving microbiological cure of *C. trachomatis*. The results of the many trials of these agents are not comparable and they can't be ranked in order of efficacy. It is, therefore, reasonable to choose on the grounds of cost, tolerability and regimen simplicity, which may affect adherence.

Where budgets allow, azithromycin offers the simplicity of a single-dose treatment that is highly effective, due partly to guaranteed adherence. Consequently, although the cost of treatment with azithromycin is considerably more than that with the alternatives, there is evidence that it is the most cost-effective. The reported cure rates of all the antibiotics listed below overlap. Although amoxicillin is not effective against *C. trachomatis* in vitro, it seems to be more effective and is better tolerated than erythromycin in pregnant women. Conversely, ciprofloxacin shows good in vitro activity but has been ineffective in clinical trials. Resistance of *C. trachomatis* to antibiotics is not widespread but has been reported. Some notes on the individual antibiotics are included in Box 2.8, but it is good practice to become familiar with the datasheet of the one or two you most frequently prescribe.

Box 2.8: Drugs used for the treatment of uncomplicated chlamydial infection

Drug	Use in pregnancy	Notes	Side effects
Azithromycin	Yes[1]	A single dose of 1 g achieves microbiological cure in 88–100% of infections in men and 91–100% of women Concentrations in the uterus and prostate have been estimated to remain above the MIC_{90} for up to 10 days The dose should be taken 1 hour before or 2 hours after food or the use of antacids	Gastrointestinal[2]
Doxycycline Minocycline	No	Cure rates 97–100% in men and 92–100% in women have been reported Doxycycline is also active against *N. gonorrhoeae* and *U. urealyticum* Once daily dosage may improve adherence, although twice daily dosage is usually recommended Milk and antacids do not affect absorption Tablets should be taken with or after food while sitting or standing and with adequate fluids to avoid the risk of oesophageal ulceration or irritation	Gastrointestinal[2] Photosensitivity Oesophagitis (rare)
Oxytetracycline Tetracycline Deteclo	No	Widely used and known to be efficacious. Inexpensive. Frequency of dosing may reduce adherence, so no longer first line Tablets should be taken with or after food while sitting or standing and with adequate fluids to avoid the risk of oesophageal ulceration or irritation Avoid milk products and antacids with dose Warnings: epilepsy, renal impairment	Gastrointestinal[2] Oesophagitis (rare)

Box 2.8: (Cont'd) Drugs used for the treatment of uncomplicated chlamydial infection

Drug	Use in pregnancy	Notes	Side effects
Erythromycin	Yes (except estolate)	Less efficacious than azithromycin or doxycycline unless given at higher doses, such as 2 g per day, or for a longer course. Gastrointestinal side effects are dose-related. A test of cure for *C. trachomatis* is recommended after treatment with erythromycin	Gastrointestinal[2] (common, dose related) QT prolongation
Ofloxacin	No	Of comparable efficacy to doxycycline. Effective in the treatment of the majority of *N. gonorrhoeae* infections It should not be taken at the same time as antacids Warning: epilepsy	Gastrointestinal Insomnia Neurological

[1]Not licensed for use in pregnancy but no report of fetal abnormalities and clinical and trial evidence of effectiveness.
[2]Gastrointestinal side effects include nausea, vomiting and diarrhoea.

CHLAMYDIAL PELVIC INFLAMMATORY DISEASE

BACKGROUND

Pelvic inflammatory disease (PID) is the most important complication of sexually transmitted bacterial infection. PID has been defined as inflammation of the uterus, fallopian tubes and adjacent structures not associated with pregnancy or operative procedures. Puerperal and post-abortal infections sometimes involve sexually transmitted pathogens but are usually considered separately. About 10% of women with untreated gonococcal or chlamydial infection will develop PID.

The morbidity, expense and social implications of PID and its further complications are massive. Much published research relates to acute symptomatic PID, which is often severe and managed on an inpatient basis. This presentation remains common but many more cases, particularly those seen in GUM, family planning or primary care clinics are mild, atypical or clinically silent. The increase in opportunistic testing for *Chlamydia* in women attending general practice or family planning clinics will reveal more cases of PID with absent or minimal symptoms and signs. Risk factors for PID are listed in Box 2.9.

Pathogenesis and clinical practice

PID is caused by infection of the endocervix with pathogens that ascend to the upper genital tract to cause endometritis, salpingitis, oophoritis and inflammation of the surrounding pelvic structures.

N. gonorrhoeae and *C. trachomatis* are both known to cause PID, and gonorrhoeal infection is responsible for a high proportion of cases where the prevalence of that infection is high.

Box 2.9: Risk factors for PID

Risk Factor	Protection
C. trachomatis or N. gonorrhoeae infection	Combined oral contraceptive use
Presence of bacterial vaginosis	Barrier contraception
Intrauterine contraceptive device (IUD) insertion	
Menstruation	
Childbirth	
Uterine instrumentation	
Vaginal douching	
? IUD in situ: probably low risk	
Age – no effect when adjusted for rates of bacterial STIs	

The prevalence of *N. gonorrhoeae* is considerably lower than that of *C. trachomatis* in women in the UK and it is likely that the biggest single cause of PID in the UK is chlamydial infection.

The proportion of PID attributable to *C. trachomatis* varies from 30% to 75%, depending on the study population. There is evidence only on acute PID presenting as an emergency, in which the prevalence of gonococcal infection was 14% in a recent British study.

The role of *M. hominis*, *M. genitalium* and *U. urealyticum* in the pathogenesis of PID is unclear. *M. genitalium* and *U. urealyticum* are implicated as causes of NGU in men. *M. hominis* and *U. urealyticum* have been isolated from the upper genital tract of women with PID and *M. genitalium* is commonly isolated from the cervix of sexually active women. Rises in serum titres of antibodies to all of these organisms have been shown to occur during acute PID, but it is not clear whether they are causal or merely markers of disease.

The bacteria associated with bacterial vaginosis (BV) (see Ch. 4) can be cultured from samples of the Fallopian tubes in up to 80% of women with PID and are thought to be an important factor in pathogenesis.

BV is more common in women with PID than in controls and may facilitate the ascent of *C. trachomatis* and *N. gonorrhoeae* from the endocervix to the upper genital tract. It is for this reason that treatment of PID includes antibiotics active against these organisms.

The pathogenesis of 'silent' chlamydial-induced tubal damage and acute, symptomatic PID is currently assumed to be the same.

CLINICAL FEATURES OF PELVIC INFLAMMATORY DISEASE

Symptoms and signs

Pelvic inflammatory disease represents a spectrum of severity from asymptomatic 'silent' disease, through minimally symptomatic infection that may be – but isn't always – chronic, to severe disease that often presents acutely. Acute pelvic inflammatory disease may present as a surgical, gynaecological or medical emergency. Research relating to the frequency and reliability of various signs and symptoms has focussed on acute disease. The sensitivity and specificity of clinical diagnosis is notoriously poor, even in the acute setting. Mild or chronic symptoms and signs can present even greater diagnostic difficulty. The slight differences between the clinical presentations of gonococcal PID (see Ch. 4), such as the increased likelihood of pyrexia, as compared to chlamydial PID, are of no use in current clinical practice. Features of mild and severe PID are given in Box 2.10.

Investigations

If diagnosis is based on the presence of clinical signs, the risk of a false-positive diagnosis is 35% and of a false-negative diagnosis is 15%. Laparoscopy improves the sensitivity

Box 2.10: Features of mild and severe PID[1]

	Mild – moderate	**Severe**
Presentation to	General practice Family planning Genitourinary medicine Gynaecology outpatient	Emergency admission: surgery, gynaecology or medicine
Symptoms	Subacute or chronic Pelvic pain (Gradual in onset, or intermittent) Backache Deep dyspareunia Dysuria Menstrual irregularity Vaginal discharge	Acute Pelvic pain (90–99%) Systemic illness Anorexia and vomiting Vaginal discharge
Signs	Lower abdominal tenderness Adnexal tenderness or mass Cervical motion tenderness Cervical discharge	Lower abdominal tenderness Adnexal tenderness or mass Cervical motion tenderness Cervical discharge Pyrexia > 38°C (50%)
Investigations	Usually a clinical diagnosis, investigations opposite may be helpful in some cases Pregnancy test if any risk Test for gonococcal and chlamydial infection[2]	FBC: Leukocytosis ESR >15 mm/hour (75%) Pregnancy test/serum HCG Pelvic ultrasound Laparoscopy Endometrial biopsy Test for gonococcal and chlamydial infection[2]
Potential differential diagnosis	Endometriosis Appendicitis Crohn's disease Irritable bowel Retrograde menstruation Functional pain	Complicated ovarian cyst Tubal ectopic pregnancy Pyelonephritis Appendicitis

[1]As the condition is a continuum, there is a considerable overlap between the features of mild, moderate and severe disease.
[2]Negative tests for *N. gonorrhoeae* and *C. trachomatis* do not exclude PID.

and specificity of diagnosis, although false negatives are still common. Histological examination of samples of endosalpinx or endometrium is better still and can be performed at laparoscopy, or more simply on outpatient endometrial biopsy samples. Neither this nor laparoscopy are recommended as part of routine clinical practice in the UK. A high index of clinical suspicion with a low threshold for empirical treatment is a common pragmatic approach.

Management

The aims of treatment in PID are to:

- resolve symptoms
- avoid immediate complications
- avert long-term sequelae.

Delay in treatment of PID has been shown to increase the risk of infertility and ectopic pregnancy, particularly in chlamydial PID. Antibiotic therapy should be initiated without waiting for the results of investigations. Most of the evidence on treatment relates to acute PID, and to inpatient management. Antibiotic therapy should be active against *N. gonorrhoeae, C. trachomatis*, Gram-negative bacteria and anaerobes. In practice, most women with PID are treated as outpatients, and there is little evidence that inpatient treatment with intravenous antibiotics is more effective than oral treatment. However, admission should be considered in certain circumstances.

Centers for Disease Control and Prevention recommendations for hospital admission with PID, from which UK guidelines are derived, include:

- severe illness
- diagnosis uncertain
- surgical emergency cannot be excluded
- pelvic abscess suspected
- patient pregnant
- patient adolescent
- patient has HIV infection
- unable to tolerate oral therapy
- no response to oral therapy
- follow-up within 72 hours not possible.

Case history

Marianne (30 years) presented with backache and deep dyspareunia of 2 months' duration. Her last period had been heavier and more painful. On bimanual examination there was marked pain on cervical movement and tenderness in the right adnexum. A pregnancy test was negative. She was treated with ofloxacin and metronidazole and symptoms improved. PCR for *C. trachomatis* on an endocervical sample proved positive. She planned to start a family in the next 3 years and was counselled regarding the possibility of infertility.

Management

- Antibiotic therapy (see Box 2.11)
- Analgesia
- Bed rest if moderate/severe
- Review after 72 hours in moderate/severe cases. Reconsider referral for further investigation, including laparoscopy, if no improvement
- All women should be seen by a health adviser for partner notification and information giving

Antibiotic therapy for PID

UK (Clinical Effectiveness Group, 2001) and US (Centers for Disease Control and Prevention, 2002) guidelines recommend that antibiotics active against *N. gonorrhoeae* are used in the treatment of all cases of PID.

The use of ofloxacin plus metronidazole as first-line therapy for outpatient treatment of PID has the advantage that most strains of *N. gonorrhoeae* in the UK are sensitive to ofloxacin. There is also evidence that it is more efficacious in the treatment of PID than the commonly used alternative of doxycycline plus metronidazole for 14 days.

Box 2.11: Treatment of pelvic inflammatory disease (level of evidence)

Outpatient therapy	1st line Ofloxacin 400 mg orally twice a day plus metronidazole 400 mg orally twice a day for 14 days (III) or Ceftriaxone 250 mg i.m. stat or cefoxitin 2 g i.m. with probenicid 1 g orally followed by metronidazole 400 mg orally twice a day and doxycycline 100 mg orally twice a day for a total of 14 days (III)
Inpatient acute/severe disease	1st line Cefoxitin 2 g intravenously twice a day plus doxycycline 100 mg orally or i.v. twice a day or clindamycin 900 mg intravenously three times a day plus gentamycin 1.5 mg/kg i.v. three times a day (III) and once apyrexial and improving metronidazole 400 mg orally twice a day and doxycycline 100 mg orally twice a day for a total of 14 days or clindamycin 450 mg orally four times a day for a total of 14 days (III)

> **Box 2.12: Complications of PID**
>
> *Complications of untreated disease*
>
> | | |
> |---|---|
> | Tubo-ovarian abscess | Rare complication of severe disease
More common in HIV-infected women
Requires surgical drainage |
> | Perihepatitis | Severe acute right upper-quadrant pain usually in the presence of symptoms of PID
Occurs in 10–20% of acute PID cases
Management is as for PID |
>
> *Late complications of treated disease*
>
> | | |
> |---|---|
> | Infertility | Rate of tubal factor infertility : 10% after one episode
20% after two episodes
30% after three episodes |
> | Ectopic pregnancy | Risk is 7–10 times that of women with no history of PID
9% of pregnancies following PID are ectopic
Ectopic pregnancy is the main cause of first-trimester maternal death in developed countries |
> | Chronic pain | Occurs in 12–75% of women, more commonly with repeated episodes
Women with a history of PID are 10 times as likely to be admitted with chronic pain as controls |

FOLLOW-UP

- Women with severe acute disease should be reviewed at 72 hours.
- All women should be seen on completion of therapy (2–3 weeks) to confirm adherence, resolution of symptoms and partner notification.

For complications of PID see Box 2.12.

Partner notification

Male partners of women with PID should be treated whether or not *C. trachomatis* (or *N. gonorrhoeae*) is isolated. If *N. gonorrhoeae* is not seen on Gram-stained slides from the female urethra and endocervix, or the male urethra, at first attendance, it is reasonable to treat a male partner solely for suspected *C. trachomatis* infection.

Standard advice is to avoid intercourse until the follow-up appointment. Women may be counselled regarding the risk of infertility following PID. See Box 2.12 and below.

PATIENT INFORMATION ON CHLAMYDIAL INFECTION AND ITS COMPLICATIONS

- The diagnosis of *Chlamydia* in a sexual partner is no indication of infidelity
- Long-term carriage of *Chlamydia* can occur in both men and women without symptoms
- Neither NGU nor chlamydial infection are thought to affect male fertility.

Workers experienced in sexual health usually play down the possibility of a partner's infidelity when discussing a diagnosis of chlamydial infection, by stressing the likelihood of long-term carriage. However, the risk of infertility was the aspect of counselling most frequently recalled by women in one study. Emphasizing the probability of long-term carriage may increase this concern, so may not always be helpful. The risk of infertility after an episode of symptomatic PID can be estimated (Box 2.12) and should be explained to women with PID. Asymptomatic chlamydial infection is thought to affect fertility, but the risk is unknown. It is not known whether treatment reduces or averts this risk.

Both men and women may have anxieties regarding a partner's reaction to the diagnosis. These may include fear of rejection, the need to disclose having had previous partners, and feelings of contamination and stigmatization. Consider these possibilities whenever counselling people diagnosed with chlamydial infection or its complications.

Further Reading

Centers for Disease Control and Prevention. Sexually transmitted diseases treatment guidelines 2002. MMWR 2002; 51 (no. RR-6): 30–32. www.cdc.gov/std/treatment/rr5106.pdf.

Chlamydia trachomatis: summary and conclusions of CMO's Expert Advisory Group. London; Department of Health: 1998.

Duncan B, Hart G, Scoular A, Bigrig A. Qualitative analysis of the psychosocial impact of diagnosis of *Chlamydia trachomatis*: implications for screening. BMJ 2001; 322: 195–198.

Guaschino S, De Seta F. Update on *Chlamydia trachomatis*. Ann N Y Acad Sci 2000; 900: 293–300.

Horner P, Owen Caul E. Clinical effectiveness guideline for the management of *Chlamydia trachomatis* genital tract infection 2002. www.bashh.org/guidelines/C4A%2009%2001c.pdf.

Management of genital *Chlamydia trachomatis* infection. SIGN Publication number 42. Edinburgh; SIGN Secretariat: 2000.

McMillan S, McKenzie H, Flett G, Templeton A. Which women should be tested for *Chlamydia trachomatis*? Br J Obstet Gynaecol 2000; 107:1088–1093.

Paavonen J, Eggert-Kruse W. *Chlamydia trachomatis:* impact on human reproduction. Hum Reprod Update 1999; 5: 433–447.

Ross JDC. Outpatient antibiotics for pelvic inflammatory disease. BMJ 2001; 322: 251–252.

Sellors J, Mahoney J, Goldsmith C et al. The accuracy of clinical findings and laparoscopy in pelvic inflammatory disease. Am J Obstet Gynecol 1991; 164: 113–120.

Sweet RL. Role of bacterial vaginosis in pelvic inflammatory disease. CID 1995; 20 (Suppl 2): S271–S275.

SELF-ASSESSMENT

A 22-year-old man consults you with a 7-day history of white urethral discharge marking his underwear and mild dysuria. His last sexual contact was 8 days ago with a regular female partner of 7 months. Three weeks ago, after a 'works night out' he had unprotected vaginal sex with a casual female partner. Examination reveals mucopurulent discharge at the urethral meatus. Microscopy of a Gram stained slide of the discharge shows 20–30 PMNLs per high power field but no Gram-negative intracellular diplococci. He is extremely anxious and there is 'no way' he will tell his partner about his 'one night stand'.

Questions
a) What is the diagnosis and your first-line treatment?
b) What would you (or a health adviser) tell him about the condition and partner notification?

His partner attends a week later with a contact slip recording the NSU diagnosis and his case number. You check the result of his *Chlamydia* LCx test prior to seeing her. It is negative. She is completely symptomless.

c) What is your management? Do you give his partner treatment? What do you tell her? Consider the advantages and disadvantages of your approach.

His partner's *C. trachomatis* test result is also negative. A month later he re-attends. He is still troubled by a discharge, present when he checks in the morning, and a shooting pain in his urethra every few days.

d) What details of the history should you explore or confirm?
e) What single investigation would you suggest?

Answers
a) The presumptive diagnosis is of non-gonococcal urethritis. Results of culture for *N. gonorrhoeae* will confirm or refute this. Results of tests for *C. trachomatis* infection will confirm whether this is chlamydial or non-chlamydial NGU. The treatment is the same in either case. Azithromycin 1 g stat or doxycycline 100 mg twice daily for 7 days would be appropriate first-line treatment.
b) NGU is inflammation of the urethra. It is often caused by *Chlamydia*. Sometimes no cause for the condition is found and it can occur 'out of the blue'. Treatment with antibiotics usually cures the condition anyway. In this case, the condition was probably triggered by sex with his casual sexual partner. Both his recent partners should be tested and treated, regardless of his test results. He should not have sex with his regular partner until a week after they have both completed treatment. He should be offered the choice of self-notification, provider notification or conditional notification. It may be helpful to talk through the diagnosis of NGU and how he might explain this to his partner. He should also be given a contact slip and written information on NGU and chlamydial infection. He can be reassured that his confidentiality will be respected

should his regular partner attend the GU clinic. If he is reluctant to give contact details he should be informed of the potential risk to his partner's health.

c) It may be useful to explore what her partner has told her about his condition. She should be offered screening for sexually transmitted infections, including *C. trachomatis*. She should be offered treatment for NSGI, because she has an approximately 20% chance of chlamydial infection, and because her partner's condition may recur if she is not treated. The reasons for giving treatment even if *Chlamydia* is not detected should also be explained. The adverse effect of this is that she may worry unnecessarily about the possibility of chlamydial infection until her own test result is available. Your own approach to this situation will depend upon your understanding of the evidence base and your own beliefs and values. The duty of confidentiality, however, is paramount.

d) Explore the nature of pain and discharge. Is it occurring all the time, or intermittently? He says there is discharge 'when he checks' in the morning. Is he stripping the urethra to check for discharge? Confirm that both he and his partner completed treatment before they resumed intercourse, and that no other partners are involved.

e) Microscopic examination of a slide of urethral material obtained after holding the urine overnight would confirm or refute persistent urethritis. If such a slide contains no PMNLs he can be reassured and advised not to check for discharge. If there is objective evidence of NGU, he may be re-treated with second-line therapy.

Vaginal discharge, bacterial vaginosis, candidiasis and trichomoniasis

3

INTRODUCTION

Discharge is a common presenting symptom in women and is usually perceived and described as a vaginal discharge. Discharge may originate from the urethra, vulva, vagina, accessory glands or cervix, but in most cases presenting symptoms don't allow differentiation of its anatomical origin. The perception of discharge is subjective and physical characteristics of vaginal discharge are a very poor predictor of underlying aetiology. Normal physiological discharge is variable in character and amount, and assessment should focus on any change in, rather than the presence of discharge. The management of women presenting with 'vaginal' discharge includes a thorough history to detail any change in the character of discharge, to identify associated symptoms and to assess risk factors for STI. Consider all possible causes including the physiological as well as sexually and non-sexually transmitted pathogens (see Box 3.1). The pathogens most often encountered are not usually regarded as being sexually transmitted and include *Candida* species and organisms associated with bacterial vaginosis (BV). Sexually transmitted pathogens that do cause discharge include *Chlamydia trachomatis*, *Neisseria gonorrhoeae* and *Trichomonas vaginalis*. In sexually active women, sexually transmitted infection may co-exist with a discharge of non-STI cause. Increased physiological discharge can occur with cyclical hormonal changes over the menstrual period, or be associated with foreign bodies or cervical glandular ectopy. Women who are worried about the risk of STI may present with a perceived change in character or amount of discharge, which after examination and microbiological testing shows no evidence of pathology.

AN APPROACH TO THE MANAGEMENT OF DISCHARGE

HISTORY

Clinical history is useful in exploring the likelihood of sexually transmitted infection, which may co-exist with or may cause discharge, but history is a poor discriminator of aetiology. In the sexual health or GU clinic, all women presenting with discharge should be routinely tested for sexually transmitted infection. In other settings, where full investigation is less straightforward, it may be omitted in some cases. The history and

Box 3.1: Causes of discharge in women

Anatomical site	Causes of discharge
Urethra	**STI** Gonorrhoea Chlamydial infection Trichomoniasis NSGI **Non-STI** Urinary-tract infection
Vulva	**STI** Herpes Syphilitic chancre Other genital ulcer syndromes **Non-STI** Candidiasis
Greater vestibular glands (Bartholin's)	**STI** Gonorrhoea NSGI
Vagina	**Physiological causes** **Non STI** Candidiasis Bacterial vaginosis B haemolytic streptococci Trichomoniasis **Others** Foreign body
Cervix	**Physiological** Glandular ectopy Pregnancy IUCD **STI** Gonorrhoea Chlamydial infection Syphilis Herpes simplex virus Non-specific genital infection (NSGI) ?*Ureaplasma urealyticum* ?*Mycoplasma genitalis* **Others** Warts Cervical polyp Cervical malignancy Allergy Endometrial lesions

clinical examination may be useful in assessing which patients should undergo, or be referred for, STI screening. Women at low risk of sexually transmitted infection, such as those with a long-term regular partner, or no recent sexual partner, can be treated 'blind' for suspected candidiasis provided:

- A sexual history has been taken
- Follow-up is possible.

Although individual symptoms and signs have low sensitivity for particular infections, a combination of vulvar itch and burning with erythema, fissures and/or a curdy, non-odorous discharge on examination has high specificity for *Candida* spp. on culture. A minority of women have such a clinical presentation.

A consultation about a discharge is often a good opportunity to discuss screening for STIs. Opportunistic testing for chlamydial infection, at least, should usually be offered to women under the age of 30 years who have not previously been tested.

Follow the approach to history taking outlined in Chapter 1. Using open followed by closed questioning, concentrate on the following areas, noting their possible significance (see Box 3.2).

Box 3.2: History taking: vaginal discharge

History	Symptom	Possible significance
Nature of discharge	Change in character or volume from usual	Asking about a change in discharge is a better discriminator than presence of discharge
	Odour	May indicate BV or trichomoniasis, or foreign body such as retained tampon
	Bloodstaining	**Usually indicates discharge has a cervical rather than vaginal origin***
Accompanying symptoms	Vulval/vaginal itch	A feature of candidiasis and trichomoniasis but rare in BV
	Dyspareunia – distinguish deep from superficial dyspareunia	Superficial dyspareunia is a feature of vulvitis
		Deep dyspareunia may indicate cervicitis and/or PID*
	Post-coital bleeding	**Cervicitis/other cervical or endometrial pathology***
	Change in menstrual cycle	**Intermenstrual bleeding or menorrhagia is a feature of PID***
	Pelvic pain	**Feature of PID***
Partners	Single longstanding regular partner	Full STI screen may not be mandatory
	Recent partner change, multiple partners	**STI risk***
	Symptomatic partner	**STI risk*** (itch, pain or erythema of the glans penis following intercourse may occur in the partner of a woman with candidiasis)

*STI screen mandatory in the presence of any of these features

Nature of discharge

- Change in character or volume from usual
- Amount, colour, consistency
- Odour (constant, or occurring after intercourse)
- Change with menstrual cycle, bloodstaining.

Physiological vaginal discharge varies in amount and character between individual healthy women and in the same individual over time. Normal discharge may increase in amount midcycle or premenstrually, or change over a longer time period due to the development or regression of a cervical glandular ectropion or age-related changes to the vaginal mucosa (Fig. 3.1).

Accompanying symptoms

- Vulval/vaginal itch, vulval pain, burning
- Lumps or swellings in the vulva or groin
- Pelvic pain, dysuria, deep or superficial dyspareunia
- Post-coital bleeding, change in menstrual cycle
- Urinary urgency or frequency, dysuria or haematuria
- Rash or ulceration.

Partners

- Recent partner change
- Multiple partners
- Symptoms in a regular male partner (e.g. dysuria, discharge or penile itch)
- Concurrent symptoms in a female partner.

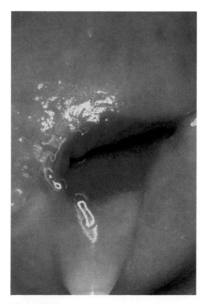

Figure 3.1
Normal cervix with clear cervical mucus

Other features

- Changes in contraceptive method (start or stop IUCD, oral contraceptive or condom use)
- Onset of symptoms relative to last sexual contact or partner change
- Onset of symptoms relating to menstrual cycle
- Anal intercourse
- Use of vaginal douche, soaps or cosmetics
- Recent antibiotic use
- Possibility of pregnancy.

Clinical notes: history taking in vaginal discharge

- Nature of discharge

- Itch or smell

- Cyclical change

- Pelvic pain

- Accompanying symptoms

- Partner change

EXAMINATION

Follow the standard examination in Chapter 1, paying particular attention to the following features, which may suggest the origin of the discharge and its aetiology (see Box 3.3).

Pubic area. Look for ulceration, excoriation, erythema or rash.

Box 3.3: Examination findings in women with vaginal discharge

Site	Examination Finding	Consider
Vulva	Excoriation, fissuring	Candidiasis
	Erythema, oedema: 'vulvitis'	Candidiasis, trichomoniasis
	Ulceration	Herpes simplex, other genital ulcer disease
	Odour	BV, trichomoniasis, foreign body
Vagina	Copious purulent discharge	Trichomoniasis, gonorrhoea, foreign body
	Curdy, white, non-odourous discharge or plaques	Candidiasis
Cervix	Ulceration	Herpes simplex, other genital ulcer disease
	Glandular ectopy with clear cervical mucus	Physiological discharge
	Inflamed cervix with mucopurulent or purulent cervical discharge	Chlamydial infection, gonorrhoea, consider PID
	Warts or polyps	May cause increased discharge in the absence of other pathogens

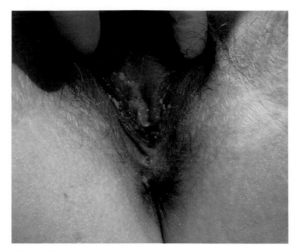

Figure 3.2
Discharge of BV at the introitus

Labia majora and minora. Note erythema, oedema, lichenification or fissuring. Discharge may be present on the labia or at the introitus (Fig. 3.2): note its colour, consistency and any odour.

Urethra and greater vestibular glands. Samples of discharge from these sites can be smeared onto a glass slide for Gram staining and microscopy.

Vagina. Look for warts or erythema. Note the colour and odour of discharge (but be aware that diagnosis based on the characteristics of a discharge can be unreliable). Be alert to the presence of a foreign body.

Cervix. Presence of normal cervical glandular ectopy, any evidence of inflammation, ulceration or genital warts. Nature, amount and colour of cervical mucus (clear, mucopurulent or purulent). The presence of cervical inflammation with yellow, purulent or mucopurulent cervical mucus indicates cervicitis.

INVESTIGATIONS

In women presenting with discharge, take a sample of vaginal discharge from the lateral and posterior vaginal fornices, smear onto a glass microscope slide for Gram staining. Take a second sample and mix with a drop of 0.9% saline on a further slide and cover with a glass coverslip. Wet-smear microscopy should be done within 10 minutes.

Test the pH of a sample of vaginal discharge from the posterior vaginal fornix or lateral wall of the vagina with a narrow range pH paper (Fig. 3.3), using either a piece of paper held in sponge forceps, a cotton wool swab, or test the discharge adhering to the speculum after removal. The pH of normal vaginal secretions, and in vulvovaginal candidiasis, is <4.5. A pH of >4.9 is indicative of bacterial vaginosis or trichomoniasis. Avoid testing the cervical mucus or lubricants, which will give a falsely alkaline reading. A sample of discharge may be mixed with potassium hydroxide (1% or 10%) on a

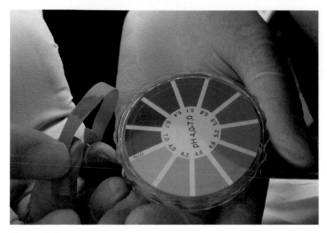

Figure 3.3
pH paper showing elevated pH in bacterial vaginosis

microscope slide to perform the amine test. The release of a 'fishy' odour is supportive of the diagnosis of bacterial vaginosis. The slide can be examined under the microscope for fungal hyphae and spores.

Culture for *Candida* species and *T. vaginalis* may be helpful in some cases but is not mandatory. Prepare cultures for *Candida* species using either Sabouraud's medium, or using a transport medium (Amies) to transfer samples to the laboratory for plating. Culture for *T. vaginalis* can be made using Diamond or Feinberg-Whittington medium, or a self-contained commercial culture kit. These kits can also be directly inoculated in the clinic, or prepared in the laboratory from an Amies swab.

BACTERIAL VAGINOSIS

BACKGROUND

Bacterial vaginosis (BV) is a common cause of abnormal discharge in women of reproductive age. The reported prevalence in women sampled in the community varies between 5% and 30% depending on geographical location and sample population. Many of these women are asymptomatic. Risk factors for the development of BV are listed in Box 3.4. In healthy women followed up over time, bacterial vaginosis may appear and resolve spontaneously. Resolution may be induced by menstruation or sexual intercourse, but intercourse can also trigger awareness of abnormal odour and precipitate consultation. The pathogenesis of BV is not fully understood but involves a depletion of the normal healthy vaginal flora and an increase in organisms including anaerobes and *Gardnerella vaginalis*. Little or no inflammation is associated with this change in flora (hence vaginosis rather than vaginitis). Although there is evidence that the same strain of *G. vaginalis* can be isolated from the urethra of a male partner as from the vagina of a

Box 3.4: Risk factors for bacterial vaginosis

Risk factor	Comment
Race	Black > Caucasian > Asian
Sexual experience	Occurs in virgins but prevalence increases in parallel with number of sexual partners
Smoking	
IUCD	
Vaginal douching	
Cunnilingus	

woman with BV, the condition is not regarded as a sexually transmitted disease. Bacterial vaginosis is implicated in the development of pelvic inflammatory disease (PID) (see Ch. 2) and women with PID have a high prevalence of BV. Although clinical experience suggests that acute pelvic inflammatory disease develops in some women immediately after the onset of symptoms of BV, there is no evidence that treating BV reduces the incidence of PID. There is currently no evidence to suggest that treatment is indicated in healthy, asymptomatic non-pregnant women diagnosed with BV. BV is an independent risk factor in the transmission of HIV, with 1.5 to 3-fold increased risk of seroconversion over matched individuals without BV in a number of prospective studies.

LABORATORY FINDINGS OF CLINICAL RELEVANCE

Lactobacilli (Gram-positive rods) (Fig. 3.4) are the predominant bacterial morphotype on Gram stained slides of vaginal secretions from healthy women.

Gram stained slides from women with bacterial vaginosis show a predominance of Gram-negative or variable rods consistent with *G. vaginalis*, small curved Gram-negative or variable rods consistent with *Mobiluncus* and Gram-positive cocci *(peptostreptococci)* (Fig. 3.5). Lactobacilli are reduced in number or absent.

Culture of vaginal fluid from women with BV (not a routine procedure) reveals a mixed colonization including *G. vaginalis*, *Prevotella* species, genital mycoplasmas, *Mobiluncus* species and others.

These bacteria adhere to exfoliated vaginal epithelial cells in large numbers and obscure the cell margin when viewed in a wet-mount preparation under dark-field microscopy (Fig. 3.6). Such epithelial cells with a granular cytoplasm and small rods evenly spaced over the cell surface, giving a stippled appearance, are called clue cells. The presence of clue cells is a sensitive test for BV. Lactobacilli do not tend to adhere to epithelial cells in the same way.

G. vaginalis is not the cause of BV per se, but appears to interact with anaerobic and other bacteria to change the vaginal environment. *G. vaginalis* is found in low concentrations in many women without BV, and if inoculated experimentally does not cause BV. Culture for *G. vaginalis* is not, therefore, a suitable test for BV.

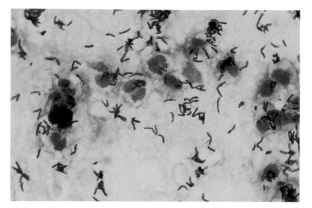

Figure 3.4
Gram stained smear of normal lactobacilli

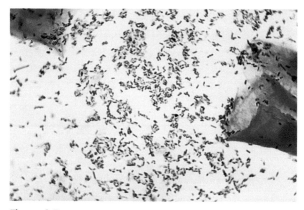

Figure 3.5
Gram stained smear of mixed organisms in bacterial vaginosis

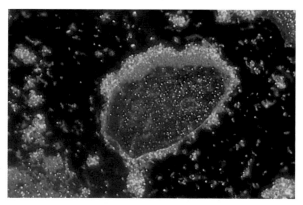

Figure 3.6
Clue cell on dark-field microscopy of wet mount of bacterial vaginosis

Proteolytic enzymes produced by anaerobic bacteria break down peptides in vaginal fluid to produce polyamines. These are thought to cause the elevation in vaginal pH associated with BV, and to produce increased amounts of volatile substances such as trimethylamine, putrescine and cadaverine that contribute to the malodour associated with the condition.

CLINICAL FEATURES

Symptoms

- None (50%)
- Odour (offensive or fishy smelling). Sometimes noted after intercourse
- Increased discharge. Discharge is rarely copious
- Pain or itch in those with BV as the only diagnosis is rare.

Signs

- Adherent white or grey discharge described as homogeneous or 'non floccular', thin (of low viscosity) and of 'milk-like consistency'
- Odour may be detectable at examination without the addition of potassium hydroxide (see below).

DIAGNOSIS

The high prevalence of BV in healthy women means that the coincidental finding of BV in women with another infection is common. Several clinical and microscopic scoring systems for the diagnosis of bacterial vaginosis have been validated. Clinical diagnosis can be made by means of the Amsel criteria. The presence of **three of the four** following is diagnostic:

- Homogeneous white adherent discharge
- Clue cells on microscopy of a wet smear (usually >20% of epithelial cells)
- Vaginal pH >4.5
- Fishy odour when mixing vaginal fluid with 10% potassium hydroxide (KOH).

Some experience of microscopy is required to identify clue cells with reliability.

Attempts have been made to produce methods of diagnosis based purely on microscopy of the Gram-stained smear. Since the 1980s, a number of systems have been validated that assess the vaginal flora by scoring the presence of various bacteriological morphotypes. They are too time consuming for use in the busy clinic but have good inter-observer and inter-centre reproducibility, so are useful for research purposes. A system described and validated by Hay and Ison uses a simpler classification to grade microscopy findings as normal, intermediate or BV. Box 3.5 compares the Nugent criteria and Hay and Ison scoring systems. These and other scoring and grading systems are designed for use in isolation from clinical criteria. However, all scoring systems include an 'intermediate' vaginal flora, including the presence of reduced numbers of lactobacilli with mixed organisms. In these cases, the presence of clinical signs and symptoms may aid diagnosis whichever method of microscopic assessment is used.

Box 3.5: Diagnosis of bacterial vaginosis

Microscopic appearance	Nugent score	Hay–Ison Grade	Diagnosis
Epithelial cells	4	0	Normal, or may be a consequence of use of intravaginal antimicrobials
Large Gram-positive rods only: Lactobacilli morphotype	0–3	I	Normal
Intermediate flora. Reduced large Gram-positive rods, small numbers of Gram-negative or variable rods	4–6	II	Intermediate The presence of supportive clinical signs can be useful
Mixed flora Gram-positive and Gram-negative bacteria and often clue cells	7–10	III	Bacterial vaginosis
Gram-positive cocci only	Not included	IV	Bacterial vaginosis

TREATMENT

Who to treat and why (grade of recommendation):

- Women presenting with symptoms (A)
- Women undergoing surgical termination of pregnancy (A) and other surgical procedures
- Some pregnant women (A).

Women with symptoms

Women presenting with typical symptoms of BV should be treated.

Some women who don't perceive their discharge as abnormal but are found to have BV feel a beneficial change following treatment. For this reason some clinicians review symptoms in women found to have BV and offer treatment. This may preclude the giving of an unequivocal 'all clear' in women presenting with concerns about STIs or a partner's infidelity, so should be done with caution. The potential adverse effects of introducing a perception of disease in well women with this common, recurrent condition have not been investigated. Although BV is implicated in the pathogenesis of acute pelvic inflammatory disease (PID), there is no evidence of a reduction in the development of PID, or PID sequelae, consequent on treating asymptomatic BV.

Surgical procedures

Treatment of BV prior to surgical termination of pregnancy has been shown to reduce the incidence of post-operative PID (level of evidence 1b). Infective complications of vaginal and of abdominal hysterectomy are higher in those with BV. Although there is no prospective trial evidence of the benefit of prophylaxis, antibiotics are usually given.

Pregnancy

BV is strongly associated with preterm birth, late miscarriage and premature rupture of membranes. Treatment of BV in pregnancy might therefore be expected to improve pregnancy outcomes. It is as yet unclear which pregnant women should be treated, when, or what with. Meta-analysis suggests that systemic antibiotic treatment of BV (usually with metronidazole) during pregnancy marginally reduces the probability of delivery before 37 weeks. Although increasing gestational age at delivery by treating infection with antibiotics does not necessarily improve neonatal or maternal outcomes, a controlled trial of the use of oral clindamycin in pregnancy showed a highly significant reduction in the rate of preterm birth. Guidelines based on current evidence do not suggest routine screening and treatment of all pregnant women, although many clinicians would now treat the chance finding of BV in an asymptomatic pregnant woman. A subgroup of women with a history of second trimester loss or idiopathic preterm birth may benefit from screening and standard systemic treatment for BV.

Case history

Jean (37 years) attended a GUM clinic having seen her GP the previous week. She had been given clotrimazole pessaries for 'thrush' to no effect. She noted that the discharge was unlike the thrush she had previously experienced. There was no itch and she mentioned an unpleasant smell, especially after intercourse. On examination there was a thin, milky vaginal discharge with pH 6.0. Microscopy showed depleted lactobacilli with many Gram-variable rods. She was treated with metronidazole 2 g in a single dose.

Antibiotic therapy

Oral metronidazole as either a single dose or a course of treatment is commonly used as first-line therapy (see Box 3.6). A course of metronidazole carries no advantage in initial

Box 3.6: Treatment of bacterial vaginosis

Antibiotic (Grade of Evidence)	Cure rate	Comments
First-line		
Metronidazole 2 g orally single dose (1a)	85% at 7–14 days,	Avoid alcohol for 48 hours after last
Metronidazole 400 mg orally twice daily for 5 days (1a)	55–75% at 4 weeks	dose. Avoid single dose in pregnancy Inexpensive
Second-line		
Clindamycin 2% cream intravaginally once daily for 7 days (1b)	60–95% at 1 month	Damages latex condoms Expensive Vulval irritation, vaginitis common
Metronidazole 0.75% gel intravaginally once (or twice) daily for 5 days (1b)	85% at 7 days	
Third-line		
Clindamycin 300 mg orally twice daily for 7 days (1b)	94% at 1 week	Occasional antibiotic colitis

(Data from Hay, 2001 and Centers for Disease Control and Prevention, 2002)

cure rate (at 1 week) over a single dose, although one of two large meta-analyses has shown a significantly better cure rate (88% vs 54%) at 4–6 weeks after treatment. This possible advantage should be balanced with tolerability of tablet taking and side effects. Oral metronidazole causes side effects including an unpleasant metallic taste in the mouth, nausea and reduced appetite in about 15% of patients. Fewer women experience side effects with single dose therapy. A disulfiram-like reaction to alcohol with metronidazole has been reported but appears to be mild and extremely rare. It is usual to recommend avoiding alcohol whilst taking therapy and for 48 hours after the last dose. Some women will find the longer period of abstinence from alcohol less acceptable than others. Most women are happy to make a choice given information on these factors.

Intravaginal clindamycin cream or metronidazole gel have comparable cure rates to oral metronidazole (1b). The use of intravaginal therapy does not seem to be associated with any significant reduction in the incidence of side effects over oral treatments, but they are useful in those women who wish to avoid oral antibiotics. Although there is good evidence (1a) that metronidazole does not cause teratogenesis in the first trimester of pregnancy, many pregnant women and their doctors opt for topical rather than systemic treatments in this circumstance. The manufacturer advises against the use of single dose metronidazole in pregnancy.

Antibiotics commonly used in the treatment of chlamydial infection or gonorrhoea (such as quinolones and azithromycin) are not effective against anaerobes. If BV is diagnosed in a woman treated, for example, as a contact of chlamydial infection, she will require metronidazole or an alternative in addition to an antichlamydial antibiotic.

INFORMATION

Reassurance that BV is not a sexually transmitted infection and carries no implication of infidelity in a regular partner is helpful (see below).

An analogy with thrush or urinary-tract infection, coming 'out of the blue' may help women who have not previously heard of the condition.

Advice against vaginal douching (evidence based) and the use of soaps and cosmetics when washing or showering (not evidence based) is usually given.

In recurrent BV it is worth exploring whether anal intercourse is practiced and advising condom use and hygiene measures, or avoiding vaginal intercourse immediately after anal intercourse.

Back up verbal information with an appropriate leaflet.

PARTNER NOTIFICATION

There is a high rate of concordance with respect to BV in monogamous lesbian couples. There is no proof of benefit of treating female partners of women with BV, but the possibility of testing and treatment should be offered.

One study has shown an association between NGU in men and BV in women. Several studies have shown no benefit in treating the male partners of women with BV, and most clinicians do not routinely screen or treat male partners of women with BV.

RECURRENT BV

Bacterial vaginosis recurs in 20–30% of women at 4 weeks, although not all of these women are symptomatic. Retreatment with the same antibiotic may be successful, although it is reasonable to use a 5-day course of oral metronidazole, or a topical treatment, after the failure of single-dose therapy. Treatment with lactobacilli or live yoghurt has not shown benefit.

VULVOVAGINAL CANDIDIASIS

BACKGROUND

Vulvovaginal candidiasis is the most commonly diagnosed cause of vaginal symptoms in women in genitourinary medicine clinics in the UK. Forty to 75% of sexually active women report one or more episodes at some time, many of which are self-diagnosed or managed in general practice. Treatment with over-the-counter preparations or empirical prescription medication is often successful. However, diagnosis on the basis of clinical signs and symptoms is unsatisfactory. One-third to one-half of women with symptoms suggesting the diagnosis do not have *Candida* spp. on microscopy or culture. The commonplace nature of the condition does not diminish its impact on the individual and symptoms of an acute episode can be severe and distressing. Recurrent symptomatic vaginal candidiasis can be particularly debilitating.

PATHOGENESIS AND CLINICAL PRACTICE

Candidiasis (or candidosis, thrush) is caused by a number of closely related saprophytic yeasts that colonize the human gastrointestinal tract. This is thought to be the source of colonization of the vagina in women.

Up to 20% of healthy non-pregnant women and 40% of pregnant women carry *Candida* species as commensal organisms in the vagina, the majority (70–90%) being *C. albicans*. Infection with other species, most commonly *C. glabrata* is clinically indistinguishable. Treatment is indicated only in those who are symptomatic.

The change from asymptomatic carriage of the saprophytic organism in blastospore form to symptomatic disease caused by epithelial invasion by growing fungal hyphae, may be triggered by several precipitating factors, but is usually spontaneous (see Box 3.7).

Of women presenting with vulvar itch and/or increased vaginal discharge, *Candida* spp. are isolated in less than one-third. Full evaluation including examination for bacterial vaginosis and testing for STIs is preferable to blind treatment.

Box 3.7: Factors implicated in vulvovaginal candidiasis

Evidence based or widely accepted association	Pregnancy Uncontrolled diabetes mellitus Immunosuppressive drugs Frequency of sexual intercourse
Anecdote, little or no evidence	Antibiotic use Tight fitting or nylon clothing Use of hygiene products
Evidence of no association	HIV infection Combined oral contraceptive New sexual partner Number of sexual partners

Candidiasis is not regarded as a sexually transmitted disease, although some men with hypersensitivity to candidal antigens may develop penile itch, balanitis (Fig. 3.7) or occasionally oedema, after intercourse with an infected female partner. Reinfection from a male partner is suspected to be the cause of recurrent candidiasis in a minority of women.

In most women with vaginal infection, the same species of *Candida* can be isolated from the rectum. Recurrence is thought to be due to re-inoculation from the gut, or from a sexual partner. However, eradicating *Candida* from the gut by using systemic antifungals, or concurrent treatment of male sexual partners, does not improve cure rates or reduce the chance of recurrence.

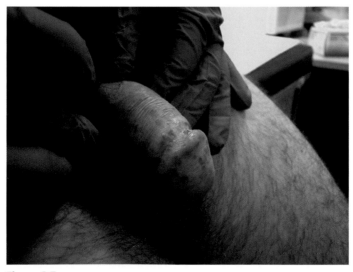

Figure 3.7
Candidal balanitis

CLINICAL FEATURES

Symptoms

- Itch (pruritus vulvae), sometimes after intercourse
- External burning dysuria
- Superficial dyspareunia
- Discharge.

Signs

- Vulval erythema and oedema (Fig. 3.8)
- Satellite lesions affecting the labia majora, the perineum, perianal region and inner thighs
- Fissuring and excoriation
- Vaginal erythema and occasionally plaques
- Thick, white, typically curdy discharge (Fig. 3.9)
- No odour.

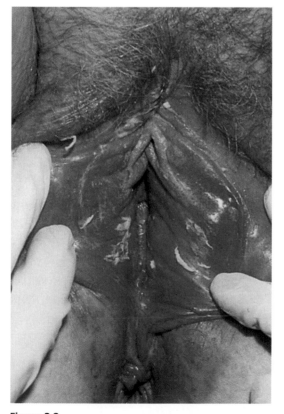

Figure 3.8
Candidal vulvitis

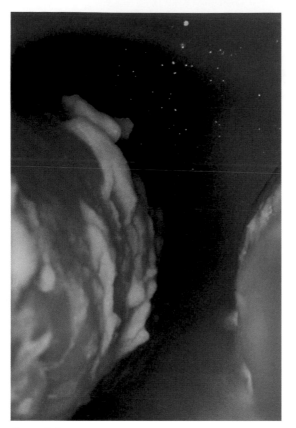

Figure 3.9
Discharge of vaginal candidiasis

DIAGNOSIS

On examination, the pH is less than 4.5 and the whiff test if performed is negative.

Microscopy of an isotonic saline wet-mount sample of vaginal discharge taken from the lateral and posterior fornices reveals spores and pseudohyphae in up to 60% of cases. A wet-mount sample prepared with 10% potassium hydroxide solution may be slightly more sensitive, but kills *T. vaginalis*, so must be done in addition to the saline wet mount if included in routine assessment of discharge.

Microscopy of Gram-stained smear of vaginal discharge may be slightly more sensitive than wet-mount examination (Fig. 3.10). Spores and pseudohyphae stain Gram positive.

Culture of samples of vaginal discharge on Sabouraud's medium is not routinely undertaken in all clinics, but is useful if symptoms and signs suggest the diagnosis, microscopy is negative and no alternative diagnosis is made. Women with vulvar symptoms and/or signs should have samples taken from the vulva during examination. These can be kept aside to be sent for culture for *Candida* spp. if vaginal wet mount and Gram stain prove negative.

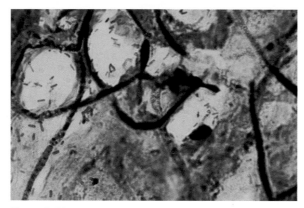

Figure 3.10
Gram-stained smear showing spores and pseudohyphae of *Candida* spp.

Fungal typing and/or azole sensitivity testing is rarely indicated and is not usually routinely available. It may be useful in recurrent vulvovaginal candidiasis or treatment failure.

TREATMENT

Clotrimazole is the mainstay of treatment, although other topical azoles including econazole, fenticonazole and miconazole are equally efficacious and should be used routinely where they can be obtained more cheaply. Nystatin pessaries are effective but a treatment course is 14 days and they are messy and less convenient than the alternatives (see Box 3.8).

Women with marked vulval irritation as well as discharge may benefit from the use of a topical antifungal cream (e.g. clotrimazole 1%) for up to 14 days after the use of a pessary. Women should be instructed in the use of the pessary/cream and applicator and advised that it will dissolve overnight leaving a residue.

Box 3.8: Treatment of vulvovaginal candidiasis

Antifungal	Cure rate	Comments
First-line		
Clotrimazole pessary 500 mg stat or 200 mg × 3 nights or 100 mg × 6 nights or clotrimazole 10% intravaginal cream	80–95%	Cheap Safe in pregnancy Sometimes disliked because 'messy'
Second-line		
Fluconazole capsule 150 mg stat orally or	80–95%	Expensive
itraconazole 200 mg bd for 1 day orally		Avoid in pregnancy and breastfeeding

(Data from Daniels and Forster, 2002, which includes many other treatment options.)

INFORMATION

- Not a sexually transmitted infection.
- Treatment of asymptomatic male partner not required.
- Usual advice is to avoid tight fitting clothing, nylon underwear and the use of soaps and irritants, though this is not evidence based.
- Some self-help books advise the avoidance of sugars, certain yeast containing foods or other dietary elements. These should be regarded with caution.
- Symptomatic male partners should be seen and screened for STI. Candidal balanoposthitis can be treated with topical antifungal cream.

Case history

Zoe (24 years) was referred by her GP to a GUM clinic having been successfully treated for thrush on six occasions in the previous year. She had marked vulvitis and *Candida* were identified on microscopy. She was treated with clotrimazole cream for 2 weeks and supplied with a clotrimazole pessary to use each month for 6 months. She underwent STI screening and was found to have asymptomatic (and unconnected) chlamydial infection.

RECURRENT OR RELAPSING VULVOVAGINAL CANDIDIASIS

Recurrent vulvovaginal candidiasis has been defined as four or more proven recurrences in 1 year. In a minority of women, history taking elicits one of the precipitating factors outlined in Box 3.7. However, the majority have idiopathic recurrent vulvovaginal candidiasis. This is now thought to be due to failure of eradication of the organism rather than re-infection.

Clinical features

- Confirm that the symptoms are due to *Candida*, not to a co-existing contact eczema or other genital dermatosis.
- Ask about history of eczema and use of perfumed soaps, douches, fabric softener and suggest avoidance.
- Ask about other medications, particularly oral steroids or antibiotics.
- Explore the timing of the symptoms. Symptoms sometimes recur at particular times, such as premenstrually, or occasionally after intercourse.
- Confirm recurrence by microscopy.
- Take samples for culture of *Candida* spp. (*C. glabrata* is less sensitive to fluconazole). Resistance testing may be indicated in difficult to treat cases.
- Test the urine for glucose.

Treatment

Choice depends on whether symptoms are recurrent or constant, their severity, the patient's feelings about long-term medication, cost and availability of medication. Many options other than those below have been described. Randomized-controlled trials of treatment versus placebo have been published, but there is no evidence to support the use of one regimen over another. Around 30% relapse after 6 months of therapy.

1. Two (or three) doses of fluconazole 150 mg 3 days apart. This increases the cure rate of recurrent candidiasis. Women with troublesome but relatively infrequent recurrences may be given a supply of treatment to keep at home.
2. A prolonged course of fluconazole 150 mg every 3 days for 2 weeks, before instituting maintenance therapy.
3. Fluconazole 150 mg orally or clotrimazole 500 mg pessary once monthly just prior to the time of symptoms, or during the second week of the cycle, increased to twice monthly if not successful, and to weekly if necessary. Alternatively, start with the higher dose frequency, reducing gradually if the patient feels confident that symptoms are controlled.
4. A 6-month course of daily or weekly therapy: fluconazole 100 mg weekly, ketoconazole 100 mg once daily, or clotrimazole pessary 500 mg once weekly.

TRICHOMONIASIS

BACKGROUND

Trichomoniasis is a common and important STI worldwide, caused by infection with the protozoan *Trichomonas vaginalis*. Evidence suggests that infection with *T. vaginalis* increases the risk of HIV transmission by a factor of four and is associated with adverse outcomes in pregnancy. In the 1970s, prevalence rates of 20–30% were reported in clinic populations studied in the UK and USA. More recent figures suggest lower prevalence, although in studies recruited from populations attending antenatal or STI clinics in Africa, or inner-city clinics in the USA, rates of infection are 20–40%. The diagnoses of candidiasis and BV are now both around ten times as common as trichomoniasis in clinics in the UK (Box 3.9), where in many centres the prevalence in GUM attendees is less than 1%. About 10 times as many women as men are diagnosed with trichomoniasis in the UK. Box 3.10 details the management of trichomoniasis in men.

PATHOGENESIS AND CLINICAL PRACTICE

T. vaginalis is a protozoan parasite with four anterior flagellae, a terminal axostyle and an undulating lateral membrane running along the side of the body. It is ovoid in shape, about the size of a leucocyte (15 microns). The organism can be seen and the moving flagellae and membrane identified in a wet-mount preparation under the light microscope, but is almost impossible to identify when fixed in a Gram stained specimen.

Box 3.9: Relative frequency of common causes of vaginal discharge, diagnosed in genitourinary medicine clinics

Diagnosis	No. of cases in women, GUM clinics, UK, 1999
Genital candidiasis	65 000
Bacterial vaginosis	60 000
Trichomoniasis	6 000

Box 3.10: Trichomoniasis in men

- Urethritis due to *Trichomonas vaginalis* infection is clinically indistinguishable from other causes of non-gonococcal urethritis.

- Balanoposthitis, prostatitis, genital ulceration, urethral stricture and infertility have also been attributed to *T. vaginalis*, though without evidence of a causal link.

- Wet-mount microscopy of urethral discharge identifies 30% of cases. The preparation of the wet mount by irrigation of the urethra with saline will improve sensitivity. A combination of wet mount of a urethral sample taken after holding the urine overnight and a centrifuged sample of early morning urine increases the detection rate.

- Culture (on specialised culture media) of both a urethral swab sample and a first voided urine specimen has the highest sensitivity.

- In practice, male partners of women with trichomoniasis are treated empirically with metronidazole.

T. vaginalis infects the urogenital tract. In women, symptoms arise from infection of the vagina causing a vaginitis, but the urethra, bladder, cervix and paraurethral glands may also be infected, so topical treatments are not curative. In men, infection of the urethral mucosa may cause a symptomatic urethritis, indistinguishable from other causes of NGU. Infection of the prostate may be symptomatic and the organism has been isolated from the epididymis and from semen.

Infection is asymptomatic in over 50% of both sexes and long term asymptomatic carriage occurs. Symptoms may develop gradually and be unnoticed, or may develop following superinfection with other organisms. The appropriate 'look back' period for partner notification has not been determined, but the incubation period in symptomatic patients was estimated to be 4–28 days.

Transmission is almost always through sexual intercourse, but non-sexual inoculation is theoretically possible. Studies in the 1950s found that *T. vaginalis* could survive for up to 45 minutes on contaminated washcloths or toilet seats. Patients may prefer to conclude that the infection was acquired in a hot tub or from a shared towel, but this should not preclude tracing of sexual partners. Vertical transmission occurs but usually resolves spontaneously.

Sixty to 100% of the female partners of men with trichomoniasis and 20–60% of the male partners of women with trichomoniasis are also infected, supporting the view that transmission occurs by sexual contact. Sexual partners of those with trichomoniasis are usually treated with antibiotics regardless of clinical findings.

After experimental urethral inoculation with *T. vaginalis*, men developed urethritis, but a minority appeared to clear the infection. Infection was found in 70% of men examined within 48 hours of sex with an infected woman, but in only 12% of those examined after 5 days. This further supports the notion of sexual transmission and of spontaneous clearance in men.

Co-infection with other organisms is common, particularly infection with the organisms associated with BV. *N. gonorrhoeae* and *C. trachomatis* are isolated in up to 30% of cases in settings where the prevalence of *T. vaginalis* is high. A full STI screen is, therefore, mandatory in cases of suspected trichomoniasis.

T. vaginalis has been independently associated with an increased risk of prematurity and low birthweight in some studies but not in others. The coexistence of bacterial vaginosis appears to have an additive or possibly synergistic effect. Trichomoniasis has been associated with increased risk of HIV transmission. Bacterial vaginosis is also implicated in this association, but the interaction between trichomoniasis and bacterial vaginosis is not yet clear.

CLINICAL FEATURES

Symptoms

- None in up to 50% of women
- Vaginal discharge (Fig. 3.11)
- Dysuria
- Itch
- Abdominal pain is thought to be rare in women with trichomoniasis alone. The suspicion of coexisting pelvic inflammatory disease in such cases should be high.

Signs

- Erythema and oedema of the vulva and vagina. Occasionally a severe vulvitis and vaginitis.
- Discharge (may be white or clear but the 'typical' frothy, purulent discharge is found in 12%).
- Odour (may be due to coexisting BV).

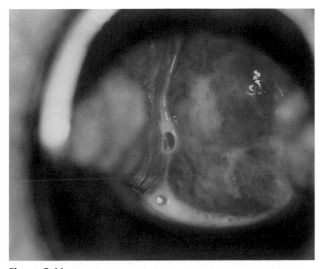

Figure 3.11
Discharge of trichomoniasis

- Strawberry cervix (colpitis macularis) visible in 2% with the naked eye and 40% at colposcopy. This finding, which describes patchy macular erythema of the cervix, is highly specific for trichomoniasis but too rare to be of routine use.

DIAGNOSIS

Wet-mount examination of a sample of material from the posterior vaginal fornix is commonly used for routine testing. An increased vaginal pH supports the diagnosis. Dark ground illumination, phase contrast microscopy or transmitted illumination at reduced intensity can be used. Sensitivity is 40–80% but cooling reduces the number of motile trichomonads rapidly from about 10 minutes after plating. Identification is largely dependent on identifying the motile protozoan and its flagellae, particularly for the inexperienced microscopist, so shouldn't be delayed.

Specialized culture media such as Diamond or Feinberg-Whittington, where available, have over 90% sensitivity. A self-contained culture system, the *In-Pouch* ™ *TV test* allows culture and repeated microscopy over several days. The system has a higher sensitivity than a combination of microscopy and conventional culture, and can be used where there are no local laboratory facilities. DNA amplification tests such as polymerase chain reaction (PCR) have been developed and are likely to become the gold standard for diagnosis in future.

Cervical cytology has a comparable sensitivity to microscopy, although in practice trichomoniasis is an incidental finding. The false-positive rate is high so the diagnosis should be confirmed by one of the above methods.

TREATMENT

Oral metronidazole in a single dose or as a course of treatment are equally effective, so a

Box 3.11: Treatment of Trichomonas vaginalis

Antibiotic (evidence level)	Cure rate	Comments
First-line Metronidazole 2 g stat (1b) or metronidazole 400 mg bd for 7 days (1b)	Cure rate 85–90% with no significant difference between regimens	Avoid alcohol Avoid single dose in pregnancy A 7 day course may reduce the chance of early reinfection and may be advisable if partner not treated concurrently
Second-line Check partner(s) treated, adherence etc Repeat 1st line (IV) or amoxycillin 250 mg tds for 5 days then metronidazole 2 g daily for 5 days (IV)	Repeat of initial therapy is usually successful	No reliable evidence on what to do in treatment failure. Many alternatives have been suggested

(Data from Sherrard, 2001 and Centers for Disease Control and Prevention, 2002)

single dose is an obvious choice (see Box 3.11). The possible disadvantages of the single dose are the slightly increased risk of nausea and vomiting, and the possibility of re-infection occurring before a partner has attended a clinic for treatment. Other notes on the use of metronidazole are as for the treatment of bacterial vaginosis.

TREATMENT FAILURE

The cure rate with a course of metronidazole is 95%. Repeated treatment failure is rare and incompletely understood.

Consider:

- Poor adherence, vomiting, re-infection
- Retreat with the same antibiotic
- Treat with amoxicillin or erythromycin prior to using metronidazole (Box 3.11) (vaginal β-haemolytic streptococci may reduce levels of metronidazole)
- High-dose metronidazole: up to 3.5 g per day orally or i.v. for up to 14 days
- Tinidazole 500 mg four times a day plus tinidazole 500 mg vaginal tablet twice a day for 14 days.

FOLLOW-UP

- Follow-up should be undertaken at 2 weeks, to confirm symptom resolution and check the results of tests for other STIs taken at first visit.
- Test of cure is not routinely undertaken unless symptomatic.
- The sensitivity of wet-mount examination is lower after treatment when trichomonads are few, so proof of treatment failure may be difficult where symptoms persist.

INFORMATION

- A sexually transmitted infection, although non-sexual transmission is theoretically possible.
- Curable and once treated there are no known long term ill effects.

SEXUAL PARTNERS

- Partner(s) should be seen, treated and offered full STI screening before further sexual intercourse.
- It is not possible to reliably exclude infection with *T. vaginalis* in men, so treatment is recommended.
- Partner notification should always include current regular partners. Evidence suggests that to offer treatment to casual partners within the last month, or the last regular partner, is also reasonable.
- The cure rate for metronidazole in the treatment of women with trichomoniasis is high even if partners are not treated, so partner notification is not ascribed the same level of importance as in other STIs.

Further Reading

Amsel R, Totten PA, Spiegel CA et al. Nonspecific vaginitis. Diagnostic criteria and microbial and epidemiologic associations. Am J Med 1983; 74: 14–22.

Bingham JS. What to do with the patient with recurrent vulvovaginal candidiasis. Sex Transm Inf 1999; 75: 225–227.

Centers for Disease Control and Prevention. Sexually transmitted diseases treatment guidelines 2002. MMWR 2002; 51(no. RR-6): 42. www.cdc.gov/std/treatment/rr5106.pdf

Daniels D, Forster G. National guideline on the management of vulvovaginal candidiasis 2002. www.bashh.org/guidelines/candida%2006%2001.pdf

Ecert LO, Hawes SE, Stevens C et al. Vulvovaginal candidiasis: clinical manifestations, risk factors, management algorithm. Obstset Gynaecol 1998; 92: 757–765.

Foxman B. The epidemiology of vulvovaginal candidiasis: risk factors. Am J Public Health 1990; 80: 329–331.

Hay PE. National guideline on the management of bacterial vaginosis. 2001. www.bashh.org/guidelines/bv_06_01.pdf

Hay PE. Therapy of bacterial vaginosis. J Antimicrob Chemother 1998; 41: 6–9.

Ison CA, Hay PE. Validation of a simplified grading of Gram stained vaginal smears for use in genitourinary medicine clinics. Sex Transm Inf 2003; 78: 413–415.

Ison CA, Savage M, Taylor-Robinson D (eds) on behalf of the Bacterial Special Interest Group of the MSSVD. Microscopy for sexually transmitted infections. London; MSSVD: 2001.

Lugo-Miro VI, Green M, Mazur L. Comparison of different metronidazole therapeutic regimens for bacterial vaginosis. A meta-analysis. JAMA 1992; 268: 93–95.

Moodley P, Connolly C, Sturm AW. Interrelationships among human immunodeficiency virus type 1 infection, bacterial vaginosis, trichomoniasis and the presence of yeasts. J Infect Dis 2002; 185: 69–73.

Sherrard J. National guidelines on the management of *Trichomonas vaginalis*. 2001. www.bashh.org/guidelines/tv%200601.pdf

SELF-ASSESSMENT

Joanne (28 years) says that she has had repeated episodes of thrush, causing severe itch, every 2 months or so since she married 4 years ago. She has 'tried everything', including giving her partner treatment. He 'keeps reinfecting her' and they are avoiding intercourse.

Questions
a) What do you wish to explore in the history?
b) How would you confirm the diagnosis?
c) What treatment and advice will you give her if candidiasis is confirmed?

Answers
a) Details of the symptoms, including itch, pain, dyspareunia. How has the diagnosis of thrush been made (is it a self-diagnosis or a clinical diagnosis)? Has the diagnosis ever been confirmed, either by microscopy or culture? Has she used treatment, if so what, and with what effect (if symptoms are not relieved quickly with treatment, consider alternative diagnoses)? If she has used multiple treatments, what did she prefer and what worked best? How do the symptoms relate to sex? Are they worse after sex, or is intercourse uncomfortable or painful? Alternatively, is she avoiding sex only because she believes that her partner is infecting her with *Candida*? How predictable is the timing of episodes, particularly in relation to menstruation? You may want to explore any predisposing causes at this stage, such as antibiotic therapy, douching, nylon underwear. Does she currently have symptoms?
b) Examine carefully for evidence of alternative diagnoses. Perform wet-mount and Gram-stained smear microscopy. Culture for yeasts either using Sabouraud's medium or an Amies swab to transport a sample to a laboratory. It may be worth taking swabs from the vulva as well as the vagina as infection can be confined to this area.
c) You may be partly guided by what she has used in the past. If she is currently symptomatic you could use a single clotrimazole 500 mg pessary plus a 2-week course of clotrimazole 1% cream applied to the vulva. If she has tried pessaries and creams without success, a course of fluconazole 150 mg every 3 days for 1 or 2 weeks may be effective. There are many alternatives – see text and Further reading. A 6-month course of maintenance therapy may be given immediately, but as recurrences seem to be relatively infrequent, it would be reasonable to try episodic therapy first – using either a single dose or a short course of topical or oral therapy for each episode, depending on how quickly and effectively symptoms are controlled. It may also be possible to time single-dose therapy with menstruation if symptoms occur at a predictable time (often in the week prior to menstruation). She should be advised that it is unlikely that her partner is reinfecting her with *Candida*, and that the condition can be controlled without the need to avoid sex.

Gonorrhoea

4

INTRODUCTION

Neisseria gonorrhoeae, also known as the gonococcus, has been recognized as the cause of urethral discharge in men and vaginal discharge in women since its identification in 1879. Most gonococcal infections involve only the mucosa of the urogenital tract, but rectal, pharyngeal and conjunctival epithelium may also be involved. Box 4.1 details the clinical presentations of gonococcal infection. In men, urogenital infections are usually

---

Box 4.1: Clinical syndromes caused by N. gonorrhoeae

Urogenital infection	
Male	Urethritis, (common)
Female	Urethritis, cervicitis (common)
Rectal infection	
Male, female	Usually with urogenital infection
Pharyngeal infection	
Male, female	Sexual transmission by fellatio or less commonly cunnilingus Usually accompanies urogenital infection
Local complications	
Male	Prostatitis, epididymitis Infection of paraphrenal glands, paraurethral glands, periurethral abscess Rarely balanitis, orchitis, median raphe abscess
Female	Pelvic inflammatory disease (10% of untreated infections) Infection and abscesses of greater vestibular and paraurethral glands (rare)
Distal complications	Disseminated gonococcal infection (DGI)
	Less than 1% of cases. Commoner in women Septic monoarthritis or polyarthritis Erythematous macular or haemorrhagic rash Meningitis, endocarditis, pericarditis, perihepatitis (very rare)
Conjunctivitis	Adult: rare Newborn: gonococcal ophthalmia neonatorum Can be prevented by prophylactic instillation of 1% silver nitrate solution or 0.5% erythromycin ointment to each eye, once, as soon as possible after delivery. Not standard UK practice.

symptomatic, a urethritis occurring in over 80% of cases. In women, genital infection with *N. gonorrhoeae* usually involves the cervix and may cause a vaginal discharge, but in 50% of women, infection is asymptomatic. Rectal infection occurs both in women and men who have sex with men (MSM), either by direct inoculation during sex with an infected partner or, in women, by autoinoculation from vaginal secretions. Rectal infection is usually asymptomatic. Pharyngeal infection, most commonly diagnosed in women and MSM, is also asymptomatic in 90% of cases. Local complications of gonococcal infection include pelvic inflammatory disease in women, and epididymitis and prostatitis in men. Distal complications such as septic arthritis, owing to disseminated gonococcal infection (DGI), may occur in both sexes, but are now rare. Conjunctival infection occurs in babies born to infected mothers but is rare in adults. The incubation period of gonococcal infection appears to have increased since the introduction of antibiotics; a greater proportion of infections are asymptomatic and the severity of symptoms in the symptomatic has reduced. This may be a survival adaptation by the organism. The current mainstay of laboratory identification of gonorrhoea is culture, which delays diagnosis for several days after presentation. Immediate diagnosis by light microscopy of Gram-stained specimens in the clinic is important in identifying cases to allow early treatment and prevent further transmission. *N. gonorrhoeae* is a highly adaptable organism and each decade brings the emergence of new antibiotic-resistant strains. The continued control of the spread of infection depends upon appropriate use of antibiotics, surveillance of antibiotic sensitivities in the population and epidemiological treatment of partners of identified cases.

NOTES ON THE EPIDEMIOLOGY OF GONORRHOEA

The incidence of gonorrhoea fell in the USA, UK and parts of Western Europe from the 1970s until the mid-1990s. In Sweden the disease was virtually eradicated, and the prospect of eradicating gonorrhoea as an endemic infection in the UK was discussed in the early 1990s. However, since 1995, the number of cases in the UK has increased year-on-year with dramatic increases in younger people in major urban centres (Fig. 4.1). Similar increases occurred in the USA from 1998. The proportion of cases diagnosed in general practice in Scotland is around one-fifth (Fig. 4.2). Rates of infection are extremely variable within populations. High rates of infection are associated with a number of inter-related factors:

1. Age: peak incidence in the UK and the USA is 15–19 years in women and 20–24 years in men.
2. Social factors: a higher incidence of infection is associated with social deprivation, being unmarried, early onset of sexual activity and urban residency. In the UK, half of the total number of cases of gonorrhoea are diagnosed in London.
3. Sexual orientation: men who have sex with men (MSM) had much higher rates of gonorrhoea than other men until the mid-1980s, when rates fell probably because men changed their sexual behaviour to reduce the risk of HIV infection. An increase in the number of cases of gonorrhoea in MSM in the UK, Europe and USA since 1997 is thought to reflect an increase in unsafe sex. This theory is supported by a dramatic increase in the rate of rectal gonorrhoea.

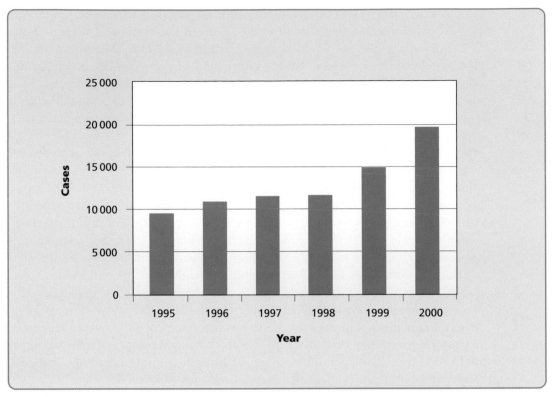

Figure 4.1
Cases of uncomplicated gonorrhoea, UK
(Data from PHLS, DHSS & PS and the Scottish ISD(D)5 Collaborative Group, 2002.)

4. Ethnicity: in both the UK and the USA, black ethnicity is associated with up to 30 × higher rates of gonococcal infection. In the UK, those of Afro-Caribbean ethnicity have the highest rates of infection, rates in those of African ethnicity are lower and rates in Caucasians are lower still. This difference is only partly explained by social factors and access to healthcare and may be due to some genetic variability in susceptibility.

5. Core groups: some people are more likely to acquire gonorrhoea and to transmit the infection in the community. They may be identified in epidemiological studies as members of a 'core group'. Core group members may be characterized by one or more overlapping social or behavioural features, such as social class, drug use, working in the sex industry or having recurrent infection. Individuals with recurrent infection are known as 'repeaters', and are diagnosed with a disproportionately large share of cases of gonorrhoea. Core group members may also include those less likely to attend for test of cure after treatment and less likely to abstain from sex when symptomatic.

PATHOGENESIS AND CLINICAL PRACTICE

N. gonorrhoeae is exclusively a human pathogen and is (almost) exclusively sexually transmitted. It is highly infectious and a single exposure infects 60–90% of females and 20–50% of males.

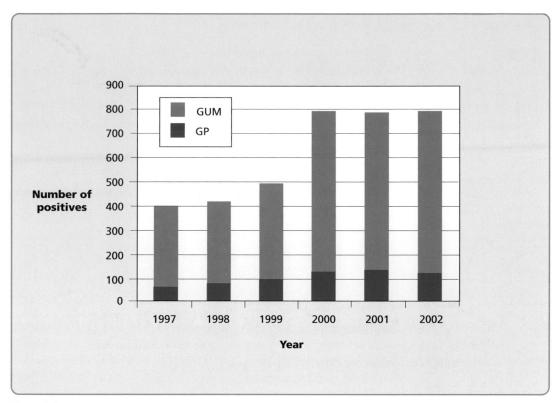

Figure 4.2
Source of positive gonococcal cultures, Scotland 1997–2002
(Data courtesy of Dr Hugh Young, Scottish *Neisseria gonorrhoeae* Reference Laboratory.)

N. gonorrhoeae preferentially infects non-cornified columnar or cuboidal epithelium. Diagnostic samples in women should, therefore, be taken from the endocervix. Vaginal samples from stratified squamous epithelium will not reliably detect *N. gonorrhoeae*.

Microscopy is unhelpful in the diagnosis of pharyngeal gonorrhoea. Other commensal organisms commonly found in the pharynx are indistinguishable from *N. gonorrhoeae*. These include *N. meningitidis,* carried in the rectum and urethra as well as the pharynx. *N. meningitidis* can be sexually transmitted, causing clinical syndromes identical to those caused by gonorrhoea (such as urethritis) in a small number of cases.

CLINICAL FEATURES

Gonococcal infections may be symptomless, particularly in women, so some people will be diagnosed with gonorrhoea at routine sexual health screens. In these cases, the diagnosis may be made only on receipt of culture results. Men and women may also present with symptoms, or as 'contacts' of gonorrhoea – that is having received a verbal or written referral to a clinic because a current or ex-partner has been found to have gonorrhoea. Diagnosis cannot be made on history alone, but certain symptoms may raise

Box 4.2: Sites of infection with Neisseria gonorrhoea *in adults*

Site	Percentage of cases infected and symptoms
Male urethra	Urethra infected in 95% heterosexual men and 60% homosexual men. >80% have discharge, 50% discharge and dysuria, 5% dysuria only
Female urethra	Urethra infected in 75%, only site infected in 5%. Dysuria uncommon.
Endocervix	Cervix infected in 90%, only site infected in 20%. Symptoms of change in discharge in up to 50%
Rectum (male and female)	Rectum infected in 40% of women (5–10% sole site of infection) and 40% of homosexual men. Symptoms in 10% include pain and discharge
Pharynx (Male and female)	Infected in 50% homosexual men, 30% of women and 15% of heterosexual men. A sore throat occurs in <20% of those infected.

the suspicion of gonorrhoea in newly presenting patients, or point to a positive diagnosis in those known to be contacts of infection. Box 4.2 details the sites infected and the likelihood of symptoms. In all cases, take a full sexual history and examine, testing for other infections as outlined in Chapter 1. In most clinics, it is not practical to perform microscopy on samples from all sites in all attendees, but factors in the presentation, history or examination may indicate which patients should undergo extended investigation. These are outlined in Figures 4.3 and 4.4.

GONORRHOEA IN MEN

History

Take a detailed history of recent sexual partners, as partner notification is a vital part of patient management. Men presenting with urethritis may be diagnosed with gonococcal or non-gonococcal urethritis (NGU) and the initial management and investigation of these conditions overlap. In gonorrhoea:

- A purulent or mucopurulent urethral discharge occurs in 80%. Dysuria and discharge together occur in 50%
- The median incubation period is 6 days
- Eighty-five per cent of men have symptoms within 14 days
- The incubation period of gonorrhoea is usually shorter than that of NGU and the discharge more likely to be purulent (see Ch. 2). However, reliable clinical diagnosis on these grounds is not possible
- Rectal infection is seen in MSM and is usually asymptomatic but causes anal discharge or pain in around 10%.

Examination

Follow the procedure for comprehensive genital examination, as outlined in Chapter 1. Routine testing for other STIs should be done in all men (10–20% of heterosexual men with gonorrhoea also have chlamydial infection). Convention dictates that examination for suspected urethritis is done at least 4 hours after last passing urine, but the optimal time is unknown.

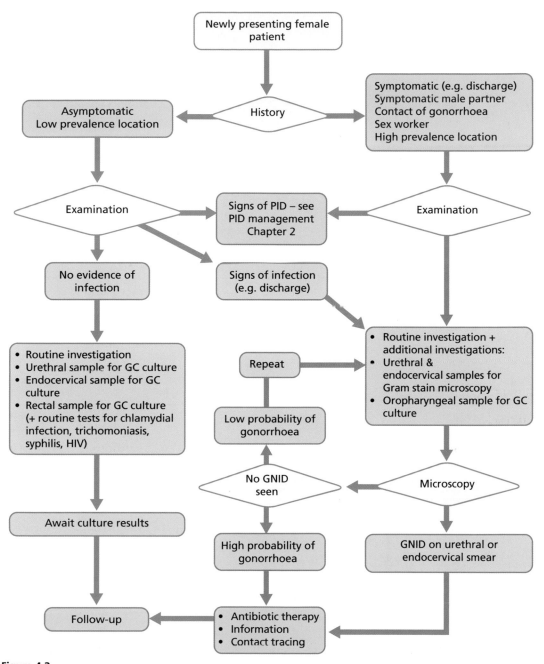

Figure 4.3
Tests for gonorrhoea in female patients

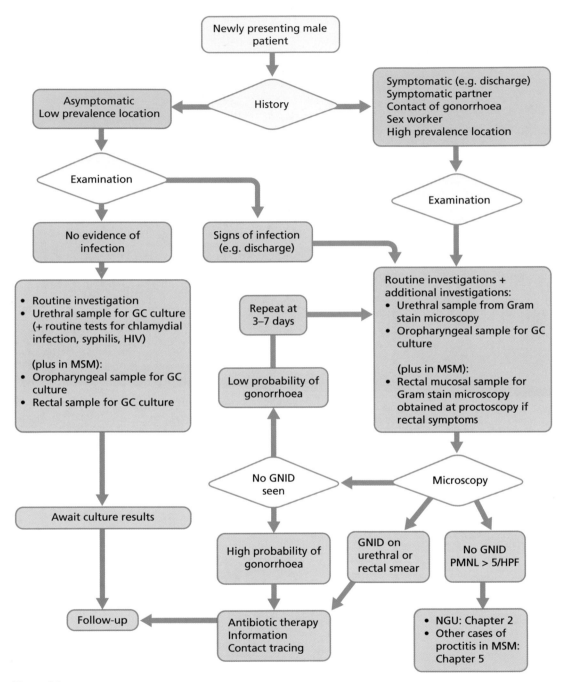

Figure 4.4
Tests for gonorrhoea in male patients

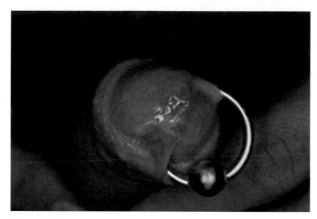

Figure 4.5
Gonococcal urethral discharge

Discharge may be visible at the urethral meatus or on the underwear (Fig. 4.5). The meatus may be inflamed.

Complications occur in only 1% of patients, but be aware of the possibility of epididymitis, septic arthritis or the rash of disseminated infection. Complications are more likely to occur in asymptomatic patients.

Men who are contacts of gonorrhoea in whom there is no evidence of urethritis should either be treated epidemiologically (see below) or examined and tested again a few days later.

Investigation

Take a sample of discharge expressed from the urethra, or from a 10 µl plastic loop inserted 2–3 cm into the urethra (Fig. 4.6). Smear onto a glass microscope slide, covering about 1 cm² for Gram staining. Take a sample for laboratory identification of

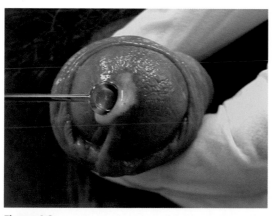

Figure 4.6
Sampling urethral discharge

Box 4.3: Sites sampled for laboratory identification of N. gonorrhoeae

	Heterosexual woman		Heterosexual man		Homosexual man	
	Routine	Contact	Routine	Contact	Routine	Contact
Throat		Yes		Yes	Yes	Yes
Urethra	Yes	Yes	Yes	Yes	Yes	Yes
Endocervix	Yes	Yes				
Rectum	Yes	Yes			Yes	Yes

N. gonorrhoeae according to the local availability of tests. If microscopy is not available on site, send the air-dried slide in a slide carrier to the laboratory.

From men who are contacts of gonorrhoea, or who have typical Gram-negative intracellular diplococci on microscopy of a urethral smear, take pharyngeal and, in MSM, rectal samples for laboratory identification.

Homosexual men with rectal symptoms should undergo proctoscopy. Take a sample of mucopus from the rectal mucosa under direct vision. Smear onto a glass microscope slide as for a urethral sample.

Box 4.3 shows anatomical sites sampled for the diagnosis of gonorrhoea.

Case history

Aidan (22 years) presented with a 3-day history of green urethral discharge and dysuria. He had been treated for gonorrhoea once before. He had two regular female partners and a casual partner 8 days previously. Microscopy of a Gram-stained urethral smear showed GNID. He was treated with a single dose of cefixime 400 mg orally. He agreed to contact both regular partners. He re-attended the clinic 3 weeks later with recurrence of discharge. *N. gonorrhoeae* isolated from his urethral swab were fully sensitive to cephalosporins. Neither of his partners had been treated. He was persuaded to return, with his partner, for simultaneous treatment. The health adviser contacted his other partner by letter.

GONORRHOEA IN WOMEN

History

Take a full sexual history as outlined in Chapter 1. Diagnosis on the basis of history is even less likely than in men. In women known to be contacts of gonorrhoea, concentrate on a full history of recent sexual contacts and symptoms suggesting upper genital-tract involvement.

- Up to 50% of all women with gonorrhoea are asymptomatic. Of women presenting as contacts of men with gonorrhoea, up to 80% are asymptomatic.
- The incubation period for gonorrhoea in women is thought to be longer than that in men, at around 10 days.
- Symptoms are non-specific and cannot be distinguished from those of other lower genital-tract infections.

- The commonest symptom is a change in vaginal discharge, originating from the infected endocervix (see Ch. 3).
- Ninety per cent of women with genital gonococcal infection have infection of the cervix.
- Seventy-five per cent of women with endocervical infection also have urethral infection, although dysuria is uncommon.
- Symptoms of cervicitis include intermenstrual bleeding, post-coital bleeding and menorrhagia. A history of pelvic pain with or without these symptoms suggests pelvic inflammatory disease.

Examination

Examination is usually normal.

- A purulent or mucopurulent cervical discharge may be seen. (In areas of high gonococcal prevalence, and/or where microscopy is unavailable, a purulent cervical discharge may be an indication for blind treatment for gonorrhoea and chlamydial infection.) The cervix may bleed easily on swabbing.
- Occasionally, a purulent discharge can be expressed from the urethra, periurethral glands or Bartholin's gland ducts. This can be smeared on a slide and Gram stained if required.
- Pelvic inflammatory disease is reported in up to 20% of women diagnosed with gonorrhoea, so have a high index of suspicion and do a bimanual pelvic examination.

Investigation

Using a 10 µl plastic loop swab inserted into the urethral meatus and a similar loop or a cotton wool-tipped swab inserted and rotated in the cervical os, take samples for Gram-stain microscopy and laboratory identification of *N. gonorrhoeae*.

Take a 'blind' rectal swab for laboratory identification of *N. gonorrhoeae*, from all women.

In women who are contacts of gonorrhoea, or who have Gram-negative intracellular diplococci on microscopy of a urethral or cervical smear, or who give a history of receptive oral sex, take a pharyngeal sample.

COMPLICATIONS OF GONORRHOEA

Pelvic inflammatory disease is the commonest complication of gonorrhoea. Other complications occur in less than 1% of cases.

Local complications

Local complications (see Box 4.1) include infection and abscess formation in glandular structures associated with the urogenital tract in men and women. Pain and swelling at the affected site, with discharge of pus from the gland orifice may progress to scarring and obstruction if untreated. *N. gonorrhoeae* does not usually affect keratinized squamous epithelium, so cellulitis is rare.

Pelvic inflammatory disease

- Gonococcal pelvic inflammatory disease (PID) is reported to develop in 5–20% of women with untreated gonorrhoea.
- The prevalence of gonococcal infection in women presenting with acute PID was 14% in a recent British study.
- Symptoms and clinical signs may be more pronounced than in non-gonococcal PID, and fever is more common. These features are not sufficiently reliable to allow diagnosis on clinical grounds.
- Microscopy of Gram-stained urethral and cervical smears has a sensitivity of 30–40%, so treatment of acute PID should include treatment for gonorrhoea.
- Management is detailed in Chapter 2.

Disseminated gonococcal infection (DGI)

The two common manifestations are the combination of fever, skin lesions and polyarthritis, or a septic monoarthritis. Other complications (Box 4.1) are very uncommon.

Skin lesions are sparse and are more noticeable on the limbs and around affected joints. Polyarthritis involves distal limb joints. Septic arthritis in a single joint, often the knee, may occur without skin lesions.

Blood cultures and joint aspirates are usually sterile, but *N. gonorrhoeae* can usually be cultured from the oral, rectal or genital mucosa of the patient or affected partner.

DETECTION OF *N. GONORRHOEAE*

MICROSCOPY

Samples from the urethra or rectum in men, or from the urethra, cervix or rectum in women, are stained with Gram's stain and examined by direct microscopy. Examine first under low power to find areas with a well-dispersed monolayer of polymorphonuclear leucocytes (PMNL). At 1000 × magnification with the oil immersion lens, the presence of typical Gram-negative intracellular diplococci gives a presumptive diagnosis of gonorrhoea. The typical appearance is of paired, small, kidney shaped, rather darkly Gram-negative staining bacteria (Fig. 4.7). There are often both intracellular and extracellular gonococci present. The cytoplasm of PMNLs may not be easily visible, but you may be able to identify diplococci lying in between the lobes of the nuclei of the neutrophil, indicating that they are intracellular. The appearance of the bacteria may be atypical in partially treated gonorrhoea, seen when patients have self-medicated with antibiotics, or those who have been treated presumptively, for example for urinary-tract infection. Inspect at least 20 fields before excluding gonorrhoea. (A definitive diagnosis requires positive **culture** for gonococcus.)

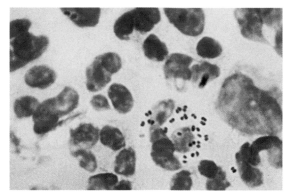

Figure 4.7
Gram-negative intracellular diplococci

Direct microscopy is sensitive in urethral samples from symptomatic male patients (89–99%), but slightly less sensitive in asymptomatic men. Microscopy of samples from the female urethra and cervix combined detects only 28–37% of genital gonococcal infections in women. This is probably due to the practical difficulties in identifying small numbers of Gram-negative intracellular diplococci in samples containing many other organisms. Similar problems exist in detecting gonorrhoea in rectal samples, which are only useful if obtained under direct vision.

Routine microscopy of samples from all clinic attendees is practiced in some clinics – particularly where the prevalence of gonorrhoea is high. In others, microscopy is restricted to those who are gonorrhoea contacts or who have abnormal symptoms or signs.

CULTURE

The isolation of *N. gonorrhoeae* by culture is still regarded as the standard method for diagnosis of infection, though this may change in the near future as nucleic acid amplification techniques such as polymerase chain reaction (PCR) and ligase chain reaction (LCR) become ever more sensitive and specific. A single set of cultures (plus direct microscopy) will detect 91–97% of infections in women. In MSM 93% of rectal infections but only 75% of pharyngeal infections are detected by a single set of cultures. In heterosexual men, asymptomatic urethral infection is rare, microscopy is sensitive and the argument against routine culture in all men can be made. However, routine urethral culture for gonorrhoea remains standard practice in the UK. Some factors to consider in choosing a culture technique:

1. Direct plating onto culture medium and immediate placing in a CO_2 incubator gives the highest diagnostic yield. This requires a regular supply of culture plates, refrigeration and an incubator. A gas storage canister with a CO_2 releasing insert (Fig. 4.8), in which plates can be transported to the laboratory is a good substitute. Medium with a shelf-life of up to a year and a built in CO_2 system has recently been developed.
2. Standard culture media consist of an enriched agar base with either horse blood, haemoglobin or serum free supplements providing amino acids and haemin. Antibiotics

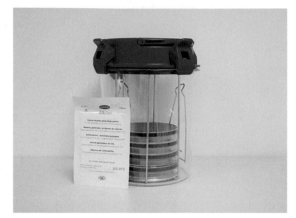

Figure 4.8
Gas jar and CO_2 producing insert for transport of culture medium to a laboratory

may be added to produce selective medium, inhibiting the growth of other commensal or pathogenic bacteria and fungi inoculated when sampling the pharynx, cervix or rectum. Thayer–Martin medium contains vancomycin, colistin and nystatin (so inhibits the growth of those strains of *N. gonorrhoeae* sensitive to vancomycin). Modified New York City (MNYC) medium contains lincomycin, colistin, trimethoprim, and amphotericin and is reported to perform better. Using selective media may potentially miss infections with strains of *N. gonorrhoeae* fully or partially sensitive to the antibiotics used. The ideal is to inoculate both a selective and a non-selective plate with a separate swab from each site. In practice this improves detection rates very little and is expensive.

3. The use of culture plates unlikely to be practicable unless a significant number of patients are to be tested for gonorrhoea at each clinic session. Samples taken from the same sites using non-toxic cotton wool swabs and placed in transport medium (Amies or an agar gel system) can be plated onto culture on reaching a laboratory. Swabs should be refrigerated at 4°C and transported to the laboratory for plating within 4 hours, after which viability deteriorates. The use of nucleic-acid testing for *N. gonorrhoeae* circumvents some of these difficulties

After 24 hours of incubation at 37°C, in moist 10% CO_2, colonies growing on culture plates are tested by the cytochrome oxidase test and if positive Gram stained for microscopy. If available, confirmatory tests include carbohydrate utilization tests, based on the ability of *N. gonorrhoeae* to metabolize only glucose, whereas other morphologically identical neisseriae metabolize other sugars including maltose and lactose. Immunological tests use monoclonal antibodies to gonococcal surface proteins to confirm identification. For epidemiological monitoring of chains of transmission or outbreaks of infection with antibiotic resistant strains, reference laboratories perform further tests allowing definitive identification of *N. gonorrhoeae* subtypes. Auxotyping identifies strains of gonorrhoea according to their requirement for specific amino acid nutrients, such as proline (P) or uracil (U). Serotyping identifies subtypes of gonococcus by the binding of specific surface proteins to a panel of monoclonal antibodies, which are then converted to a numerical code. The highest level of discrimination between gonococcal strains is achieved by opa-typing. This is a PCR method of identifying a gene so rapidly variable that similar opa-types are isolated only from sexual partners or in very short chains of transmission.

NUCLEIC ACID AMPLIFICATION

Nucleic acid amplification tests (NAAT) have been used for the detection of gonorrhoea. LCR and PCR tests can be used on first voided urine and urethral, endocervical or vaginal swabs. Sensitivities reported in several studies are 95–100% for first voided urine or urethral swabs in men and 84–95% for cervical swabs in women, with specificity of 99–100%, when compared to culture. Some, but not all studies report lower sensitivity in female urine samples. The tests appear to be highly sensitive in detecting rectal and pharyngeal infection. A higher population prevalence of gonorrhoea is detected by the use of LCR, suggesting that the test is more sensitive than culture.

Clinical notes: management of gonorrhoea

- Detailed partner history
- Gram-stained microscopy of urethral, endocervical, rectal specimens
- Culture of samples from all sites at risk of infection
- Antibiotic choice according to site and place of acquisition, knowledge of resistance patterns
- Contact tracing
- Follow up and test-of-cure

TREATMENT

PRINCIPLES OF TREATMENT

The management of the patient with gonorrhoea has implications for the individual and for the control of infection in the community. Patients diagnosed with or suspected to have gonorrhoea should usually be referred to a GU clinic or other specialist STI service for management. Treatment for gonorrhoea is given when Gram-negative diplococci are seen at microscopy, before definitive diagnosis by culture or the results of antibiotic sensitivity tests are available. This is intended to reduce the chance of transmission of infection to other partners and the development of complications.

Choosing the right treatment for gonorrhoea depends upon knowledge of patterns of in vitro antibiotic sensitivity in strains prevalent locally, the likely source of infection, the site of infection, pregnancy, tolerability, adherence, cost and any history of adverse reaction. An antibiotic is regarded as acceptable if it has been proven to eradicate infection from all sites in over 95% of cases in a trial of a size sufficient that the lower 95% confidence limit is >90%. Many antibiotics fulfil these criteria, at least for genital infection. However, endemic and sporadic resistance to antibiotics varies with location and over time, so it is not possible to recommend one antibiotic for universal use.

The successful treatment of gonorrhoea in the individual and the control of infection in the community depends upon:

1. Choosing antibiotic treatment in each individual case by predicting the likely sensitivity of the organism according to the mode and place of acquisition.
2. Rapid diagnosis, immediate treatment and high rates of successful contact tracing.
3. Follow-up and test-of-cure in all patients to detect re-infection and treatment failure in the individual.
4. In vitro culture and sensitivity testing in a high proportion of cases, including where initial diagnosis is by NAAT, to detect cases in which the infection is resistant to the antibiotic chosen, and to guide changes in prescribing policy according to local prevalence of resistance.

Choice of antibiotic

N. gonorrhoeae has shown remarkable adaptability since the introduction of antibiotic therapy in the 1940s. Strains newly resistant to the drugs used appear with regularity. Most recently a dramatic rise in the prevalence of gonococcal isolates resistant to ciprofloxacin has been seen. See Box 4.4 for details of antibiotic resistance.

Single-dose therapy for gonorrhoea is used extensively, although no oral agent has consistently shown a cure rate of over 95% in a single dose used for pharyngeal infection.

No one antibiotic will be appropriate for use in every patient in any one clinic. Protocols for first-line treatment and alternatives for infections in particular circumstances can be

---

Box 4.4: Antibiotic resistance in N. gonorrhoeae

Penicillin	High level penicillin resistance is due to plasmids carrying TEM1 beta lactamase, thought to originate from *Haemophilus influenzae* and was first identified in 1976. These penicillinase-producing *N. gonorrhoeae* (PPNG) are now distributed worldwide.
	Chromosomally mediated resistant *N. gonorrhoeae* (CMRNG), are caused by gene mutations at multiple loci affecting cell wall permeability. Penicillins are no longer recommended as first-line therapy for gonorrhoea in many parts of the world, but are still used in the UK. A regimen including penicillin, clavulanate and probenicid is effective against PPNG but not CMRNG.
Ciprofloxacin	High-level resistance to ciprofloxacin was first reported in South Asia in 1995 and is now detected worldwide. It is chromosomally mediated and resistant strains are selected by the use of low treatment doses, prompting the suggestion that higher doses should be used routinely. Fifty per cent of strains resistant to ciprofloxacin in the UK are also PPNG. The overall prevalence of ciprofloxacin resistance in the UK rose from 2.1% in 2000 to 9.8% in 2002.
Ceftriaxone Cefotaxime Cefuroxime Cefixime	Mutations causing chromosomally-mediated penicillin resistance also result in a reduction in sensitivity to cephalosporins. High level in vitro resistance to ceftriaxone has been reported in China but was not widespread in 2003.
Spectinomycin Tetracyclines	High level resistance to other antibiotics occurs. Tetracycline resistance is common: tetracyclines are not recommended as therapy for gonorrhoea. Spectinomycin resistance has not been reported in the UK or USA.

developed according to knowledge of local patterns of resistance. Box 4.5 shows the recommended regimens for the treatment of gonorrhoea. Box 4.6 gives some details on the antibiotics used.

Box 4.5: Treatment of uncomplicated gonorrhoea

First-line	Ceftriaxone 250 mg single intramuscular injection or cefixime 400 mg single oral dose[1] or cefotaxime 500 mg single intramuscular injection or spectinomycin 2 g single intramuscular injection
Second-line (if local prevalence of resistance <5% and follow-up is possible)	amoxyicillin 3 g plus probenicid 1 g single oral dose[2] or amoxyicillin 3 g plus clavulanate 250 mg plus probenicid 1 g single oral dose[2] or ciprofloxacin 500 mg single oral dose

[1]Not licensed for single dose treatment of gonorrhoea in the UK.
[2]Not recommended by CDCP and suitable only in settings outlined in text.
(Modified in the light of 2003 resistance data from Bignell, 2001 and Centers for Disease Control and Prevention, 2002.)

Box 4.6: Drugs used for the treatment of gonorrhoea

Drug	Use in pregnancy	Notes	Side effects Cautions
Penicillins: Amoxycillin Ampicillin	Yes	Always given with probenicid to delay renal excretion and give a sustained high plasma level. High failure rate in oropharyngeal infection (40–60%) Inexpensive, well tolerated, but high level resistance limits use.	Hypersensitivity
Cephalosporins: Ceftriaxone Cefotaxime Cefixime	Yes	Usually given as IM injection. Very high efficacy (96–100%) in a single dose, including oropharyngeal and rectal infection. Painful injection. Expensive. Cefixime can be given orally but unlicensed as single dose therapy for gonorrhoea in the UK. Limited evidence suggests it is as effective as injected cephalosporins. Some justification for reserving these agents for use in serious (non-STI) infections, but suitable where origin of infection unknown, adherence poor, follow-up unlikely.	Hypersensitivity (in 10% of those penicillin sensitive)
Fluoroquinolones: Ofloxacin Ciprofloxacin	No	First-line single-dose therapy until 2003 in UK, but increasing resistance means no longer recommended. Should not be taken at the same time as antacids. Warning: epilepsy.	Gastrointestinal Neurological Caution: seizures

The use of a penicillin as first-line therapy continues in parts of the UK and may be appropriate where other aspects of management are executed to a high standard. A penicillin can be used in cases where local prevalence of PPNG is less than 5%, infection is thought to be acquired locally, genital infection only is likely (so not in MSM or sex workers) and sensitivity testing and/or follow-up for test of cure is available.

N. gonorrhoeae with resistance to first-line antibiotics were isolated in 10% of infections in the UK in 2000. An antibiotic to which the organism is sensitive cures >95% of infections, intermediate 85–95% and resistant <85%. Resistance does not, therefore, automatically equate with treatment failure and a reliable test-of-cure is an alternative to using another antibiotic.

Figure 4.9 suggests a workable approach to antibiotic choice and test-of-cure based on national and international guidelines and standard UK practice. It is by no means the definitive approach, but you are likely to 'overtreat' rather than 'undertreat' infection by following it.

Co-infection with Chlamydia trachomatis

Co-infection with *C. trachomatis* occurs in 15–40% of cases of gonorrhoea in heterosexual men and women. The options are to treat for possible co-infection at gonorrhoea diagnosis, or to review with the result of a test for chlamydial infection. Factors that influence this decision are shown in Box 4.7.

COUNSELLING, INFORMATION AND PARTNER NOTIFICATION

INFORMATION

Information on gonorrhoea and its implications should be given. If a provisional diagnosis is made on microscopy, this should be made clear, even though false positives

---

Box 4.7: Factors to consider in treating possible co-infection with C. trachomatis

Await test results ⟵	⟶ Treat for possible *C. trachomatis*
Men (co-infection less common, serious sequelae uncommon)	Women (co-infection common, serious sequelae common)
Homosexual men (because of above)	Heterosexual men (because of above)
Attendance for follow-up likely	Attendance for follow-up unlikely
Single traced partner	Multiple partners
Will abstain from intercourse	Won't abstain from intercourse
Age > 30 (low rate of chlamydial infection)	Age < 30 (high rate of chlamydial infection)
High sensitivity test for *C. trachomatis* available	High sensitivity test for *C. trachomatis* not available

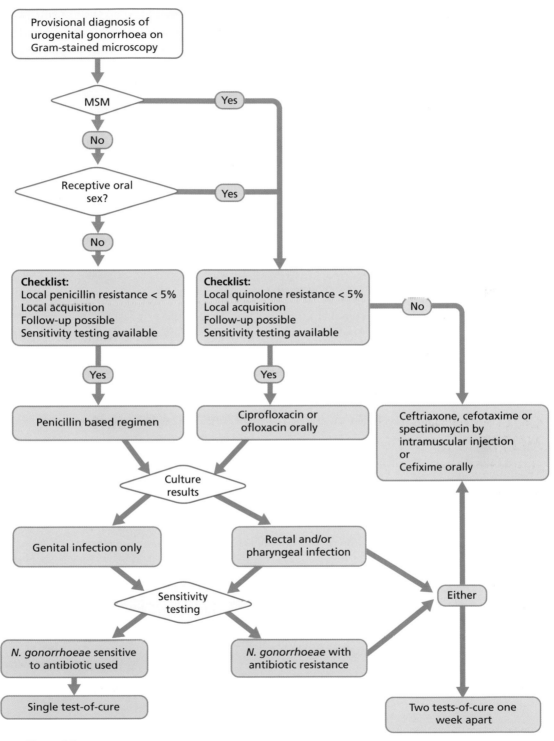

Figure 4.9
Antibiotic choice and test-of-cure in the management of gonorrhoea

are rare. If treatment for possible chlamydial infection is given simultaneously, the reason for this should be explained. The importance of treatment of partner(s), particularly female partners, should be detailed. Reinforcing advice with written information in the form of a leaflet is best.

PARTNER NOTIFICATION

From European Guideline on the management of gonorrhoea and 2001 CEG Guideline on the Management of Gonorrhoea in Adults:

- Men and women with symptoms: all partners in the last 2 weeks or the last sexual partner should be notified (because the majority of people who develop symptoms of gonorrhoea do so within 2 weeks of infection)
- Asymptomatic men and women: all partners in the last 3 months or the last sexual partner should be notified.

Treatment of contacts of gonorrhoea

People identified as contacts of gonorrhoea by partner notification may be tested for infection and treated only if positive, or treated in advance of diagnostic test results. The latter option – epidemiological treatment – is now recommended in most settings. Epidemiological treatment 'may be given when the clinician considers that the risk to the patient of unnecessary treatment is outweighed by the risk of complications of the infection or the probability of transmission of the infection to other contacts'. In deciding whether to give epidemiological treatment in the individual case, consider:

- The prevalence of gonorrhoea in sexual partners of men and women diagnosed with infection is 40–90%. In the UK in 1995 the rate was 60% in women and 75% in men
- Ten to 20% of women with gonorrhoea develop PID and this seems likely to occur early in the course of infection

---

Box 4.8: Treatment of complicated gonococcal infection

Epididymitis	See Ch. 5, Box 5.3
Infection of local glandular structures in men and women	Treat as epididymitis
Pelvic inflammatory disease	See Ch. 2
Disseminated gonococcal infection	Ceftriaxone 1 g intravenously (i.v.) or by intramuscular injection (i.m.) every 24 hours or cefotaxime 1 g i.v. every 8 hours followed by ciprofloxacin 500 mg orally every 12 hours or ofloxacin 400 mg orally every 12 hours

(Evidence level IV for all treatments)
(Data from Bignell, 2001 and Centers for Disease Control and Prevention, 2002.)

- Diagnosis by microscopy is sensitive only in male urethral infection. Microscopy will miss up to 70% of infections at other sites. A single culture will fail to detect 25% of pharyngeal infections. If epidemiological treatment is not given, two sets of negative cultures are required to reliably exclude infection.

All patients who receive treatment should be screened for STI and see a health adviser to discuss partner notification. If culture results are positive, test-of-cure should be undertaken and partner notification completed in the usual way.

FOLLOW-UP

Where resources allow, all patients should have post treatment cultures following treatment for gonorrhoea. This is particularly important where full antibiotic sensitivity testing is not routinely performed.

Arrange for follow-up at least 72 hours after treatment, when a test-of-cure can be taken. All sites initially culture positive should be re-tested.

Patients with infection of the rectum and particularly the pharynx have a higher chance of treatment failure. Detection of gonorrhoea from these sites is also less reliable. Optimal management is, therefore, to perform two tests-of-cure following treatment; the first at 72 hours to detect drug resistance, a second at 7–10 days to exclude re-infection and allow treatment of co-existing chlamydial infection.

In modern practice a single follow-up appointment at about 2 weeks is pragmatic. Test-of-cure can be undertaken, health advice can be reinforced and contact tracing can be completed.

Further Reading

Bignell C. National guideline on the management of gonorrhoea in adults. 2001. www.bashh.org/guidelines/gc%200601.pdf

Bignell C. Antibiotic treatment for gonorrhoea – clinical evidence for choice. Genitourin Med 1996; 72: 315–320.

Carne CA. Epidemiological treatment and tests of cure in gonococcal infection: evidence for value. Genitourin Med 1997; 73: 12–15.

Centers for Disease Control and Prevention. Sexually transmitted diseases treatment guidelines 2002. MMWR 2002; 51(no. RR-6): 36–40. www.cdc.gov/std/treatment/rr5106.pdf

Ison CA. Antimicrobial agents and gonorrhoea: therapeutic choice, resistance and susceptibility testing. Genitourin Med 1996; 72: 253–257.

Low N, Sterne JAC, Barlow D. Inequalities in rates of gonorrhoea and chlamydia between black ethnic groups in south east London: cross sectional study. Sex Transm Inf 2001; 77: 15–20.

Moran JS and Levine WC. Drugs of choice for the treatment of uncomplicated gonococcal infections. Clin Infect Dis 1995; 20 (Suppl 1): S47–65.

Nicoll A, Hamers FF. Are trends in HIV, gonorrhoea and syphilis worsening in Western Europe? BMJ 2002; 324:1324–1327.

PHLS, DHSS & PS and the Scottish ISD(D)5 Collaborative Group. Sexually transmitted infections in the UK: New episodes seen at genitourinary medicine clinics, 1991–2001. London; Public Health Laboratory Service: 2002.

SELF-ASSESSMENT

A 23-year-old gay man attends your clinic for the first time complaining of discharge from his anus and pain when passing stools. He has no urethral discharge, no abdominal pain and no systemic symptoms. His last sexual contact was 6 days previously with a regular male partner of 2 months. He had unprotected receptive and insertive peno-oral and oro-anal sex, and protected receptive anal sex. His partner now has a urethral discharge.

Questions

a) Outline further details you might explore in the history, the examination and tests taken.

He has had oral sex only with three casual partners in the last 2 weeks, all in the UK and from the UK. He had unprotected receptive anal sex with his regular partner 2 weeks ago, and on a few other occasions. Gram-stain microscopy of urethral smear reveals few pus-cells but no GNDC. Gram-stain microscopy of pus obtained from the inflamed rectal mucosa at proctoscopy reveals mixed organisms including extracellular GNDC, but no intracellular GNDC.

b) Should he be treated for gonorrhoea? If so, with what and why?
c) What other issues should be addressed in his immediate management?
d) How should he be followed up?

Answers

a) The immediate problem, previous risk of other STIs and future risk of STI must be addressed.

History: other partners? Open or closed relationship? Safety agreement (agreement on what sex takes place outside the relationship). Previous sexual partners. Recent travel. Hepatitis A and B testing and vaccination status. Last HIV test, if ever, and result. Condom use (always or sometimes, condom type, use of lubricants, condom slips/breakages). Recreational drugs during sex.

Examination: full systemic examination including skin, oral cavity and genital examination. Urethral samples for Gram-stain microscopy, for gonococcal identification and testing for chlamydial infection. Throat sample for gonococcal identification. Proctoscopy and swabs from rectal mucosa for microscopy for gonorrhoea, gonococcal identification, testing for chlamydial infection, and for isolation of herpes simplex virus. Testing for hepatitis A antibody, hepatitis B core antibody (anti-HBc) and hepatitis B surface antigen (HBsAg) unless history of vaccination (see Ch. 8). Offer HIV testing after full HIV pre-test discussion.

b) The most probable cause of his rectal symptoms and discharge is gonorrhoea. The development of urethral symptoms in his partner supports the diagnosis.

Immediate treatment is appropriate. There is a high probability of pharyngeal infection and a significant possibility of penicillin resistance. Treatment with a penicillin or quinolone-based regimen is not the preferred option, but could be used if sensitivity testing and follow-up for test-of-cure was guaranteed.

Successful treatment is more likely with an oral or injected cephalosporin. He may be reluctant to agree to treatment with an injectable antibiotic, especially without a definitive diagnosis. The use of oral cefixime, although unlicensed, is a possible alternative.

c) His partner should be seen and examined without waiting for culture confirmation. An attempt should be made to trace casual partners.

Consider starting a course of vaccination against hepatitis B and hepatitis A (the alternative is to wait for results of serological tests). He should be advised to abstain from sex until his regular partner has been treated and culture results are available. STI risk including HIV both within the relationship and with casual partners should be discussed. (Unprotected anal sex, carrying the highest risk of HIV transmission, is more likely to occur between men in regular relationships than with casual partners.)

d) He should be seen at least once to confirm the diagnosis, resolution of symptoms, abstention from sex and that his partner has been seen in a clinic. If culture and sensitivity testing reveals gonorrhoea sensitive to the antibiotic used, test-of-cure is not mandatory but would be usual in UK practice.

Other conditions associated with the sexual transmission of infection

5

INTRODUCTION

Epididymitis in men, pelvic inflammatory disease in women and reactive arthritis are conditions that sometimes occur as complications of sexually transmitted infection. In the UK, pelvic inflammatory disease is commonly (in 15–65%) associated with chlamydial infection, and less commonly with gonorrhoea. It is considered with chlamydial infection in Chapter 2. Although acute prostatitis is sometimes seen as a complication of gonorrhoea, it is much more commonly attributable to organisms associated with urinary tract infection. There is little evidence to suggest that chronic prostatitis is associated with STI, but it often causes genital or pelvic pain and urinary tract symptoms, and, consequently, presents in the sexual health clinic. Sexually acquired reactive arthritis is a seronegative arthropathy triggered by chlamydial infection and occasionally other STIs.

A variety of enteric infections not usually regarded as STIs may occur in men who have sex with men (MSM) as a result of sexual transmission.

PROSTATITIS

Prostatitis is rarely caused by sexually transmitted infection. Acute prostatitis is a relatively rare but serious condition associated with urinary pathogens in which diagnosis and treatment is often straightforward. Chronic bacterial prostatitis (CBP) is also uncommon, but conditions causing pelvic pain in men, previously referred to as prostatitis, are not. Chronic prostatitis is an incompletely understood condition sometimes associated with infection that presents difficulties in diagnosis, definition and management. Psychological factors may result from or precipitate physical symptoms and the management of men with chronic prostatitis requires a holistic approach to care from the outset. Consistency, explanation and support are required as, in a significant proportion of cases, no cure can be offered.

TERMINOLOGY

The developing but still incomplete understanding of the aetiology and pathogenesis of prostatitis is reflected in changes in classification and terminology. A 1995 classification, by the U.S. National Institutes of Health, divides clinically apparent prostatitis into:

- Acute bacterial prostatitis
- Chronic bacterial prostatitis (CBP)
- Chronic pelvic pain syndrome (CPPS) (inflammatory) – previously known as chronic abacterial prostatitis
- CPPS (non-inflammatory) – previously known as prostatodynia.

In acute prostatitis bacteria are usually isolated from the urine. In CBP bacteria are isolated from the prostatic fluid. In CPPS (inflammatory), excess numbers of inflammatory cells but no bacteria are found in the prostatic fluid and in CPPS (non-inflammatory) neither excess inflammatory cells nor organisms are found.

PATHOGENESIS AND CLINICAL PRACTICE

Acute prostatitis is caused by bacterial infection of the prostate gland. Bacteria isolated from the urine include *Escherichia coli*, *Pseudomonas aeruginosa*, *Klebsiella* spp. and *Proteus* spp. Gonococcal prostatitis is rare in the developed world and prostatitis rarely occurs as a complication of sexually transmitted infection. Histological findings in acute prostatitis are typical of bacterial infection, with a neutrophil infiltrate, hyperaemia and micro-abscesses.

The same organisms are implicated in the pathogenesis of CBP but are isolated from the prostatic fluid rather than the urine. CBP is regarded as a complication of urinary-tract infection, although the absence of concurrent urinary tract infection should be demonstrable in order to make the diagnosis. The involvement of urethral organisms such as *Ureaplasma urealyticum* in CBP is unclear. Histological examination of the prostate reveals similar but less marked inflammatory changes, fibrosis, microabscesses and calculi.

The pathogenesis of CPPS is ill-understood. Bladder neck abnormalities and urinary reflux have been demonstrated, and myalgia and referred pain have been implicated. Microorganisms including *Chlamydia trachomatis* and *Ureaplasma urealyticum* have been suggested as causal, but there is little evidence to support their role in pathogenesis. More recently, workers have identified elevations of pro-inflammatory cytokines in CPPS. It seems likely that psychological factors are a component in at least some cases.

CBP and CPPS are diagnosed and classified by the lower urinary tract localization procedure first described by Stamey. It is not clear whether the distinction between inflammatory and non-inflammatory forms of the condition as discriminated by his procedure relate to different pathogenic processes. Differentiation between different types of chronic prostatitis rarely affects clinical management.

ACUTE PROSTATITIS

CLINICAL FEATURES

Symptoms

Symptoms of acute onset may occur with or following those of urinary tract infection:

- Urinary tract symptoms: frequency, urgency, dysuria

- Febrile symptoms: fever, arthralgia, myalgia
- Prostatic pain: perineal, suprapubic, low back and penile pain. Pain tends to be less of a feature of acute prostatitis than of chronic prostatitis. Symptoms of urinary outflow obstruction, including acute retention of urine, may occur as a result of prostatic swelling.

Signs

Examination reveals systemic signs of infection including fever and tachycardia. Palpation of the prostate by per rectum examination reveals an extremely tender, slightly swollen, warm, tense and irregular prostate. A systemic examination will exclude other foci of infection. Prostatic massage should not be undertaken – it may precipitate bacteraemia.

INVESTIGATIONS

Microscopy and culture for gonorrhoea should be performed along with routine testing for other STIs, although *N. gonorrhoeae* is rarely implicated. A mid-stream sample of urine should be sent for culture and sensitivity testing, making the laboratory aware of the possible diagnosis and the need for sensitivity testing on any organism isolated. Full blood count and blood cultures should be taken from men with severe systemic illness.

Case history

Gordon (40 years) complained of dysuria at the start and end of his urinary stream for 5 days. Over the last 3 days he had developed low back and perineal pain, fever and rigors and increasing urinary frequency. Prostatic examination was almost impossible due to extreme tenderness. His urine contained +++ of blood on dipstick testing. He was treated with ciprofloxacin 500 mg bd for 28 days and made a complete recovery.

TREATMENT

Antibiotics should be started immediately. Consider i.v. therapy for those with symptoms of bacteraemia. Men who are treated as outpatients should be advised to reattend promptly if they fail to improve. Recommended antibiotic therapies are shown in Box 5.1.

Box 5.1: Treatment of acute prostatitis

Oral therapy	Ciprofloxacin 500 mg twice daily for 28 days or ofloxacin 400 mg twice daily for 28 days or trimethoprim 200 mg twice daily for 28 days
Parenteral therapy	Ceftriaxone, cefotaxime 500 mg single dose plus gentamicin 4 mg/kg/day until improved, then oral therapy as above.

(Data from Walker and Wilson, 2001.)

CHRONIC PROSTATITIS

BACKGROUND

The name chronic prostatitis remains in use as the umbrella term for conditions causing chronic pelvic pain in men, although the presence of inflammation of the prostate in many cases is questionable. In a small proportion (about 5%) of symptomatic men, there is evidence of bacterial infection and the diagnosis is CBP. In men with no evidence of infection, the term CPPS is probably more helpful to the patient and the clinician. The population prevalence of symptoms consistent with CPPS has been estimated to be 2–3% from studies in Canada and the USA. In the UK such men are cared for by GPs, urologists and genitourinary medicine physicians. CPPS remains ill-understood and neither diagnosis nor any of the many treatments attempted to date are supported by conclusive evidence.

Case history

Dave (38 years) presented with several months of pain in the tip of his penis, lower back and perineum. He also had pain on ejaculation. His GP had treated him empirically with azithromycin, then prolonged courses of doxycycline and ciprofloxacin. When seen in the GUM clinic he was off work, avoiding sex and his mood was low. Investigation showed no evidence of urethritis or urinary-tract infection. A lower urinary-tract localization procedure was not performed. He was treated with terazosin 2 mg, the dose increasing over 2 weeks, and referred to a clinical psychologist. He had improvement but not resolution of his symptoms. He returned to work and resumed his sex life.

CLINICAL FEATURES

Symptoms

Genital pain involving the penis, perineum, suprapubic and inguinal regions, testes and abdomen, and occasionally low back pain are features of both CBP and CPPS. Urinary frequency, urgency and changes in urine flow, and pain on ejaculation may also feature. Recurrent episodes of pain and urinary symptoms with episodes of complete relief are typical of CBP, whereas persistent, fluctuating symptoms persisting for many months or years suggest CPPS. Unfortunately, symptoms are not sufficiently clearly distinguished to allow diagnosis on clinical grounds. The chronic and possibly multifactorial nature of the condition, means that a comprehensive history at first attendance is important. The impact of the condition on everyday life, work and relationships, mood and psychological factors, and the patient's thoughts about the problem should be explored.

Examination

A full examination and testing for sexually transmitted infections is indicated as outlined in Chapter 1. It is important to exclude the possibility of NGU, as many of the symptoms are similar. Arrange for examination to take place at the time of an early morning smear (see Ch. 2), so the possibility of NGU can be excluded without the need for repeat visits. If necessary, a lower urinary-tract localization procedure can be performed at the same

> *Clinical notes: history taking in chronic prostatitis*
>
> ■ Pelvic pain: penis, abdomen, testes, perineum, back
> ■ Urinary symptoms: dysuria, frequency, incomplete emptying
> ■ Ejaculatory pain
> ■ Symptoms of urethritis
> ■ Timescale of symptoms
> ■ Relapse and remission
> ■ History of urinary-tract infection (?confirmed on culture)
> ■ Relationships, sexual function
> ■ Psychological effect of symptoms
> ■ Work and recreation.

time. Examination is not otherwise helpful as the prostate may or may not be tender on examination.

INVESTIGATION

In all patients:

- STD screen
- Gram-stain microscopy of a urethral smear
- Mid-stream sample of urine for microscopy and culture.

In men over 40 years:

- Serum prostate-specific antigen.

In men with predominantly urinary symptoms, haematuria or haematospermia:

- Flexible cystoscopy.

Other investigations sometimes used:

- Semen culture
- Transrectal ultrasound
- MRI prostate.

The lower urinary-tract localization procedure may be used to differentiate between different forms of chronic prostatitis. It involves obtaining a first voided and mid-stream sample of bladder urine, a sample of expressed prostatic secretions by prostatic massage and a post-massage urine sample. Microscopy of the secretions and quantitative microscopy and culture of the urine samples allow differentiation of urethritis, UTI, CBP and inflammatory and non-inflammatory forms of CPPS. It is a well-established procedure and no definitive diagnostic method is available to replace it. However, its utility and validity in clinical practice have been questioned for a number of reasons:

1. The distinction between CBP and CPPS may be useful in identifying patients with CBP involving bacteria associated with UTI. However, many clinicians give a trial of treatment with antibiotics even if no bacteria are isolated.

2. There is little evidence for a difference in pathogenesis between CPPS–inflammatory and CPPS–non-inflammatory, and no clear difference in the appropriate treatment.
3. The procedure is time consuming for the doctor and uncomfortable for the patient.
4. There is no correlation between findings and symptom severity and evidence of prostatic inflammation is common in asymptomatic men.

The procedure requires close co-operation between the local microbiology laboratory and the clinic. It is a procedure probably best confined to use in tertiary referral centres by clinicians with a special interest in the condition and isn't described in detail here.

TREATMENT

Antibiotics are the first-line treatment of choice in both CBP and CPPS. It has been suggested that the success of antibiotics in the treatment of CPPS is related to anti-inflammatory properties rather than any antibacterial effect. In CBP diagnosed on microbiological culture, the choice of antibiotic can be made on the grounds of sensitivity. However, in most cases in clinical practice, this is not possible. In a systematic review of treatments Collins (2000) concluded that the evidence does not support any particular treatment approach. A possible approach is described in Box 5.2.

PATIENT INFORMATION

Whatever medication is given, an important part of management is explanation of the condition and the management plan. Regular ejaculation for prostatic drainage has sometimes been advocated as part of treatment. Certainly addressing any effect on sexual relationships is important. Simple reassurance that sexual transmission isn't implicated may help, but more proactive intervention may be required where the condition has interfered with sexual function. Encouraging return to normal activity, particularly work and sports can also be useful. In some cases, the help of a clinical psychologist or couples counsellor should be sought.

Partner notification is not required.

Box 5.2: Treatment of CBP/CPPS

First-line	Ciprofloxacin 500 mg twice daily for 28–90 days or doxycycline 100 mg twice daily for 28–90 days Explanation of the condition. Reassurance regarding sexual transmission. Encourage gradual return to normal function.
Second-line	Terazosin 2 mg daily, increasing to 10 mg for 28–42 days or alfluzosin 2.5 mg three times daily for 28 days Consider stress management, cognitive behavioural therapy, psychological assessment depending on symptoms.
Third-line	Choices include non-steroidal anti-inflammatory drugs, pollen extract, acupuncture, low-dose amitriptyline, gabapentin and others.

Follow-up

Monthly appointments are justified while taking medication, in order to review progress and side effects and reinforce information giving. Patients with chronic pelvic pain are sometimes regarded as 'heart-sink' patients in GUM and urology practice, but ongoing support may help the patient to cope with the condition.

ACUTE EPIDIDYMITIS

BACKGROUND

Acute epididymitis may be due to sexually transmitted infection or may be associated with organisms causing urinary-tract infection. The likelihood of sexually transmitted cause is related to age: men under 35 years are more likely to have epididymitis due to *C. trachomatis* or *N. gonorrhoeae*. The majority of men over 35 years presenting with acute epididymitis are likely to be infected with Gram-negative enteric bacteria associated with urinary-tract infection, or following bladder surgery or cystoscopy. Sexual transmission of coliforms occurs in men who are the insertive partner in unprotected anal intercourse, usually men who have sex with men. Orchitis may be clinically indistinguishable from acute epididymitis: it occurs as a complication of systemic viral and bacterial infections including mumps, tuberculosis and syphilis.

EPIDEMIOLOGICAL AND LABORATORY FEATURES OF CLINICAL RELEVANCE

Local bacterial infection including STI usually affects predominantly the epididymis; epididymitis. The testis may be involved to a lesser degree and the condition is then termed epididymo-orchitis. The terms are used virtually interchangeably.

Chlamydial infection has been found to be responsible for the majority of cases in younger men in developed nations, even in studies using low-sensitivity tests such as enzyme immunoassay (EIA) or culture, which probably underestimate the rate of chlamydial infection. The proportion of cases due to gonococcal infection is proportional to the prevalence in the community. The role of other organisms, including *Ureaplasma urealyticum* and *Mycoplasma genitalium* is subject to debate along similar lines to that over the aetiology of non-gonococcal urethritis.

In men over 35 years, the organisms isolated include *E. coli*, less commonly *Klebsiella* and *Pseudomonas* spp. Infection with coliforms causes a more destructive epididymitis with abscess formation. This may be reflected in a higher frequency of scrotal erythema and swelling and a higher complication rate in these cases.

CLINICAL FEATURES

The most important aspect of clinical assessment is the distinction between acute epididymitis and testicular torsion. A gradual onset over several days, dysuria or urethral discharge and the presence of fever and urethritis on examination supports a diagnosis of epididymitis. Onset over a few hours, younger age (especially <20 years), lack of fever and a highly placed transverse testis within the scrotum supports testicular torsion. However, the diagnosis is not always clear and any diagnostic uncertainty should be resolved using either colourflow Doppler examination or surgical exploration. This should be organized immediately, as the viability of a torted testis is closely related to the promptness of surgical correction.

Take a sexual history in all cases of testicular pain.

Symptoms

- Unilateral testicular pain
- Fever
- Chills
- Dysuria.

Signs

- A swollen, tender scrotum, usually unilaterally
- Erythema of the scrotal skin
- Signs of urcthritis
- Hydrocele.

Men with testicular pain may have urethritis only. Men with pain, no evidence of urethritis and no tenderness on examination should be referred for surgical review.

INVESTIGATION

Perform a full set of tests for sexually transmitted infections, including Gram-stain microscopy to identify urethral gonorrhoea or non-gonococcal urethritis. At least half of all men with epididymitis have clinical evidence of urethritis, although most do not have symptoms. Obtain a urine sample for culture.

The 'two-glass' urine test may prove useful in the assessment of epididymitis: threads or cloudiness in the first sample only suggests a urethritis, usually caused by STI. Threads may also be extracted for Gram-stain microscopy (see Ch. 2). Cloudiness of both samples, sometimes with microscopic haematuria, is associated with coliform infection.

Checklist: investigation of testicular pain

- Gram-stained urethral smear
- Test for *C. trachomatis*
- Culture for urethral *N. gonorrhoeae*
- Mid-stream urine sample for microscopy, culture and sensitivity
- 'Two-glass' urine test
- Colourflow Doppler examination

Box 5.3: Treatment of epididymitis

Indication	Regimen (level of evidence III for all treatments)
Sexually transmitted infection suspected, men under 35 years	Ceftriaxone 250 mg i.m. single dose or ciprofloxacin 500 mg orally single dose plus doxycycline 100 mg orally twice daily for 14 days
Enteric organisms suspected, allergic to cephalosporin or tetracyclines, or over 35 years	Ofloxacin 200 mg or 300 mg twice daily for 14 days

(Data from Walker and Wilson, 2001.)

MANAGEMENT

- Antibiotics (Box 5.3)
- Scrotal support
- Bed rest
- Non-steroidal anti-inflammatory drugs.

COUNSELLING, INFORMATION AND PARTNER NOTIFICATION

Information

Men should be advised to reattend if symptoms deteriorate. Sexually transmitted epididymitis usually resolves within 2 weeks but mild pain and swelling may persist for several more weeks, and thickening of the epididymis on the affected side may be perceptible indefinitely.

Partner notification

Men with microscopic evidence of urethritis or suspected sexually transmitted infection should be advised to abstain from intercourse until partner(s) are seen and treated. The partners of all men under 35 years old with epididymitis and negative urine cultures, regardless of the results of STI testing, should be offered testing and/or epidemiological treatment for chlamydial infection.

Follow-up

Review at 3 days. If there is no evidence of significant improvement, reconsider the diagnosis and request a surgical opinion. The possibility of missed testicular torsion, abscess, infarct, orchitis or most importantly testicular neoplasm must then be considered.

SEXUALLY ACQUIRED REACTIVE ARTHRITIS

BACKGROUND

Sexually acquired reactive arthritis (SARA) is one of the group of spondyloarthropathies affecting the axial skeleton and non-articular structures that are triggered by environmental agents in people with a genetic predisposition. In developed countries reactive arthritis (RA) usually occurs as a rare complication of urethritis, usually associated with chlamydial infection. In developing nations the same spectrum of disease also commonly occurs as a result of enteric infection. Box 5.4 shows the organisms that trigger reactive arthritis. An aseptic arthritis occurs within 1 month of the initiating infection, accompanied by one or more of conjunctivitis, enthesitis, mucocutaneous lesions and rarely carditis. In reactive arthritis triggered by enterobacteria, urethritis may occur as part of the syndrome. The triad of urethritis, conjunctivitis and arthritis is known as Reiter's syndrome, but variations of the condition without all three features are commonly seen. The pathogenesis of *Chlamydia*-induced arthritis is a rapidly developing field and the definition and classification of reactive arthritis is likely to change as understanding increases.

PATHOGENESIS AND CLINICAL PRACTICE

SARA is triggered by infection with *C. trachomatis, U. urealyticum and M. genitalium*. It is clinically similar to the reactive arthritis seen following shigella dysentery, salmonellosis and possibly respiratory infection with *Chlamydia pneumoniae*. It is not clear whether reactive arthritis follows infection with *N. gonorrhoeae,* or whether reactive arthritis reported in cases of gonorrhoea reflects undetected chlamydial infection.

C. trachomatis has very rarely been cultured from affected joints and the condition has traditionally been regarded as a reaction to prior infection. However, there is increasing evidence that metabolically active aberrant forms of *C. trachomatis* may persist in synovial tissue. It is also suggested that the production of the powerful immunogen HSP60, also implicated in the pathogenesis of trachoma and PID (see Ch. 2), is upregulated in persistent infection. These factors may explain why antibiotic therapy for acute chlamydial infection appears to reduce the likelihood of development of reactive arthritis, whereas treatment of enteric infections does not.

Box 5.4: Bacteria that trigger reactive arthritis

- *Chlamydia trachomatis*
- *Salmonella* species
- *Shigella flexneri*
- *Yersinia enterocolitica*
- *Campylobacter fetus jejuni*
- *Clostridium difficile*
- *Chlamydia pneumoniae* (unconfirmed)

(Modified from Khan MA, 2002.)

CLINICAL FEATURES

Symptoms occur within a month of an episode of urethritis. Reactive arthritis is reported at least ten times as frequently in men as in women. This may represent underdiagnosis in women with asymptomatic chlamydial infection who present with seronegative arthritis.

HISTORY

Symptoms of the main manifestations of the disease should be explored:

- Urethritis: discharge and dysuria are often the first symptoms
- Oligoarthritis: acute onset of pain, stiffness and swelling in the affected joints. Usually asymmetrical, lower limb, affecting in order of likelihood knees, ankles and toes. Hand and finger involvement are also common
- Cystitis: usually mild, but occasionally haemorrhagic
- Sacroiliitis: low back or iliac pain, worse at night, sometimes radiating to the groin
- Enthesitis: inflammation of the ligament insertions manifesting as Achilles tendonitis and plantar fasciitis, occasionally causing pain in the sole of the foot
- Conjunctivitis (in one-third) presenting as irritation and rarely anterior uveitis, involving uniocular pain and visual disturbance
- Rash: patients may complain of a red, painless rash on the penis (circinate balanitis) or brownish thickened skin on the soles of the feet or elsewhere (pustular psoriasis/keratoderma blenorrhagica)
- Systemic symptoms.

A full sexual history should be taken, plus any history of treated asymptomatic chlamydial infection and family history of seronegative arthritis.

Examination:

- Head-to-toe systemic examination should be performed in every suspected case
- Skin: firm, dark red papules and pustules of pustular psoriasis on any part of the skin surface (Fig. 5.1)
- Eyes: mild conjunctival inflammation is common. The irregular, partly obscured pupil of anterior uveitis may be seen
- Mouth: pale, painless macules on the buccal mucosa and geographical 'bald patches' on the tongue (Fig. 5.2)
- Hands: dactylitis ('sausage digits'), small joint arthritis, onycholysis
- Cardiovascular system: (rarely) signs of myocarditis or pericarditis
- Joints: one or more affected joints are swollen and red with evidence of an effusion and limitation of movement. Tenderness over the sacroiliac joints
- Genitals: painless psoriatic lesions of the shaft or glans penis, or circinate balanitis of the glans (Fig. 5.3). Urethral inflammation and discharge. Cervicitis in women
- Feet: thick walled, brown bullae on the soles of the feet (keratoderma blenorrhagica) (Fig. 5.4). Tenderness on deep palpation due to plantar fasciitis.

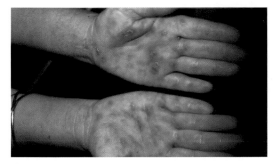

Figure 5.1
Keratoderma blenorrhagica of palms

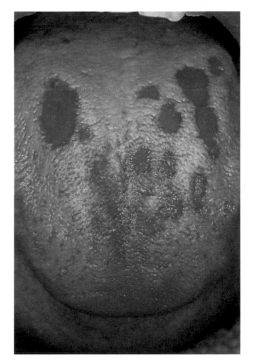

Figure 5.2
'Bald' mucosal lesions of the tongue

Investigation

The extent of investigation required depends on the severity of the condition and the certainty of the diagnosis. As a minimum:

- Microscopy of a Gram-stained urethral smear (to confirm urethritis and exclude gonococcal infection)
- Screen for sexually transmitted infections
- Full blood count, ESR (mild neutrophilia and ESR >50 mm/hour).

113

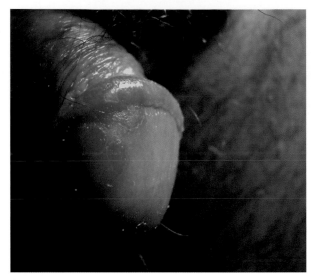

Figure 5.3
Circinate balanitis

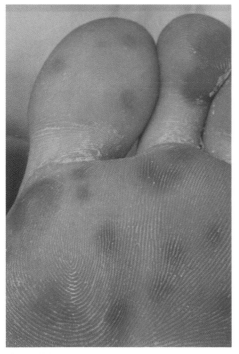

Figure 5.4
Keratoderma blenorrhagica

Where the diagnosis is less clear or symptoms are more severe, further investigations should be considered, usually in conjunction with a rheumatologist who can advise on further management. Further investigation is outlined in Box 5.5.

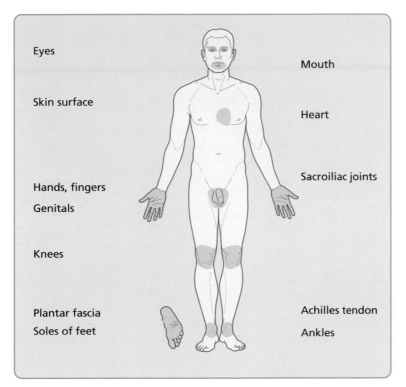

Examination Box 5.1 Clinical notes: Examination in SARA

Box 5.5: Investigations in SARA

Indication	Investigation
Other triggers of reactive arthritis	Stool culture
Differential diagnosis	Throat and rectal swabs, joint aspiration (gonococcal arthritis) Blood culture (septic arthritis) Rheumatoid factor (seropositive arthritides) *Borrelia burgdorferi* titres (lyme disease) Urate and pyrophosphate (gout and pseudogout) HIV Ab, HepBsAg, EBV titres (viral arthritis)
Disease severity	HLA B27 (recurrence more likely) Urinalysis (renal involvement)
Complications	Slit-lamp examination Joint X-rays ECG Echocardiograph

COUNSELLING, INFORMATION AND PARTNER NOTIFICATION

Information

The need for bed rest and time off work to aid recovery should be stressed. The likely duration of illness (3–5 months) and the likelihood of mild joint symptoms persisting for up to a year after this should be discussed. Recurrence occurs in 15–30% and may be triggered by a further episode of infection. It is much more likely in those who are HLA B27 positive. Recurrence usually takes the form of arthritis without non-articular involvement, though anterior uveitis does occur. Patients (especially if known to be HLA B27 positive) should be advised on the avoidance of further infections, through safer sex and hygiene, especially when travelling. They should seek prompt treatment of urethral symptoms or enteritis, as there is evidence that this reduces the chance of recurrent arthritis.

Partner notification

Advise to abstain from intercourse until partner(s) are seen and treated.

Partner notification is as for uncomplicated chlamydial infection (Ch. 2).

Follow-up

Review mild cases until arthritis settles, there is no evidence of complications and contact tracing is confirmed. Moderate and severe cases should be followed up by a rheumatologist.

TREATMENT

The condition is usually self-limiting and there is no cure. Symptoms last on average 3–5 months and 15–30% have mild chronic symptoms in the year following. In mild cases, treatment of the triggering urethritis and simple analgesia is effective (Box 5.6). Corticosteroids and immunosuppressants are used in moderate to severe disease. At

---

Box 5.6: Management of sexually acquired reactive arthritis

Mild disease	Treat urethritis (azithromycin or doxycycline)
	Regular aspirin or ibuprofen in standard doses, indomethacin if required
	Topical steroid for plasma cell balanitis (e.g. betnovate)
	Topical steroids for conjunctivitis (e.g betamethasone eye drops)
	Bed rest
Moderate/severe disease or second-line therapy	As above plus
	Shared care with rheumatologist, ophthalmologist
	Physiotherapy
	Corticosteroid joint injections
	Oral corticosteroids
	Azathioprine, methotrexate, sulphasalazine, gold
	Anti-TNF α therapy

present, there is some evidence that treatment of chlamydial infection with antibiotics may affect the likelihood of SARA occurring, but there is no conclusive evidence that the duration of therapy or the antibiotic used influences the course of the disease. Treatment of urethritis should, therefore, be with standard therapy (Ch. 2).

SEXUALLY ACQUIRED ENTERIC INFECTIONS

BACKGROUND

Men who have sex with men (MSM) may present with symptoms of proctitis due to rectal infection with sexually transmitted organisms. Enteric organisms causing proctocolitis or gastroenteritis may be transmitted through oro-anal contact (Box 5.7). Organisms such as *Cryptosporidium* spp. that cause a self-limiting illness in immunocompetent men, but a more severe and sustained diarrhoeal illness in men with HIV, may also be sexually transmitted. The prevalence of intestinal protozoa in homosexual men is 10–30%. Many of these men are asymptomatic and routine screening for intestinal pathogens is not required.

CLINICAL FEATURES

Sexually transmitted pathogens may cause a proctitis. The proctitis of chlamydial infection or gonorrhoea is commonly mild and asymptomatic. In a minority of cases there may be rectal pain, tenesmus and blood or slime on the stools. The proctitis of initial episode herpes infection may be extremely severe.

Symptoms of proctocolitis accompany infection with bacterial enteric pathogens such as *Salmonella* and *Shigella*. The symptoms, investigation and treatment of these enteric organisms are the same as when transmitted by the oro-faecal route (Box 5.8) and are not considered in further detail here.

Box 5.7: Gastrointestinal and rectal symptoms in MSM

Sexually transmitted infections	*N. gonorrhoeae* *C. trachomatis* Herpes simplex virus *Treponema pallidum*
Enteric pathogens	*Campylobacter* spp. *Shigella* spp. *Entamoeba histolytica* *Giardia intestinalis* *Cryptosporidium* spp. Coronavirus
Other causes	HIV infection Inflammatory bowel disease Irritable bowel syndrome Trauma

Box 5.8: Investigation and treatment of enteric infections in MSM

Organism	Symptoms (may be asymptomatic)	Diagnosis	Treatment
Shigella spp.	Diarrhoea	Stool culture	Supportive Antibiotic if severe and known sensitivity
Campylobacter spp.	Diarrhoea, abdominal pain, anorexia	Stool culture Serology	Supportive Erythromycin 500 mg twice daily for 5 days
Cryptosporidium spp.	Watery diarrhoea, abdominal pain, vomiting	Stool microscopy (Z-N statin) Rectal or small bowel biopsy	Supportive
Giardia lamblia	Bloating, flatulence, anorexia, nausea	Stool microscopy Jejunal aspirate	Metronidazole 2 g daily for 3 days
Entamoeba histolytica	Diarrhoea, flatulence (rarely right upper quadrant pain due to hepatic abscess)	Microscopy of faeces or material from rectal ulcer	Metronidazole 800 mg three times daily for 5 days, then diloxanide furoate 500 mg three times daily for 10 days

Investigation

Screen for sexually transmitted infections in other sites, as outlined in Chapter 1.

Do proctoscopy, looking for evidence of erythema, bleeding and pus on the rectal mucosa. Occasionally discrete ulceration is seen. The differential diagnosis includes herpes, syphilis and *Entamoeba histolytica* – although non-invasive amoebae are a common finding in homosexual men and are indistinguishable from *Entamoeba histolytica* on microscopy. Take swabs under direct vision, from areas of pus or ulceration if seen, for:

- Gram-stained smear microscopy for *N. gonorrhoeae*
- Identification of *Chlamydia trachomatis*
- Herpes simplex virus identification.

Take stool samples for microscopy to identify ova, cysts and parasites.

If cultures prove negative and symptoms persist, further stool samples should be examined. Additional investigations occasionally required include rectal biopsy, colonoscopy and small bowel biopsy.

TREATMENT

Specific treatments for sexually transmitted infections are described in the appropriate chapters. Supportive therapy including fluids, electrolyte solutions and rest are given in all cases of proctocolitis with diarrhoea. Antibiotic therapy is usually reserved until microscopy or culture results are available.

COUNSELLING, INFORMATION AND PARTNER NOTIFICATION

Contact tracing for sexually acquired enteric infections is as for genital infection. There is no evidence to guide contact tracing in men with enteric infection. Regular partners should probably be offered investigation. Food handlers and care workers should be advised regarding employment. Cases of *Salmonella*, *Shigella* and *Campylobacter* should be notified to the local Department of Public Health.

Further Reading

Collins M, MacDonald RMS, Wilt TJ. Diagnosis and treatment of chronic abacterial prostatitis: A systematic review. Ann Intern Med 2000; 133: 367–381.

Inman RD, Whittum-Hudson JA, Schumacher HR, Hudson AP. Chlamydia and associated arthritis. Curr Opin Rheumatol 2000; 12: 254–622.

Khan MA. Update on spondyloarthropathies. Ann Intern Med 2002; 136: 896–907.

Luzzi GA. Chronic prostatitis and chronic pelvic pain in men: aetiology, diagnosis and management. J Eur Acad Dermatol Venereol 2002; 163: 253–256.

Luzzi GA, O'Brien TS. Acute epididymitis. BJU Int 2001; 87: 747–755.

McMillan A. Intestinal and anorectal disorders in homosexual men. In McMillan A, Young H, Ogilvie MM, Scott GR (eds). Clinical practice in sexually transmissible infections. Edinburgh; Saunders: 2002.

O' Mahoney C. The diagnosis and management of prostatitis. In: Barton SE, Hay P (eds). Handbook of genitourinary medicine. London; Arnold: 1999.

Walker P, Wilson J. 2001 National guideline for the management of epididymo-orchitis. www.bashh.org/guidelines/epididymoorchitis%200601.pdf

Walker P, Wilson J. 2001 National guideline for the management of prostatitis. www.bashh.org/guidelines/prostatitis%2006%2001.pdf

SELF-ASSESSMENT

Alan (22 years) is referred to the genitourinary medicine clinic with a pain in his right knee. He noticed some urethral discharge about 3 weeks ago and some slight dysuria and backache on a couple of occasions last week. The pain began to develop over the last 4 days and he missed football training 2 days ago. It became more severe yesterday afternoon and worsening through the evening. He is now 'in agony'.

Questions
a) What other aspects of the history are important?
b) What are the two main differential diagnoses in this man?
c) Considering the differential diagnoses, what factors on examination might influence your choice of investigations.

He has a non-gonococcal urethritis, ESR 65 mm/hour and mild neutrophilia. Other immediate investigations are non-diagnostic. He is systemically well.

d) What is your management?

Answers
a) Other symptoms including fever, chills and malaise that might suggest a septic arthritis (they are relatively uncommon in SARA). Ask about pain or swelling in other joints. Low back pain, pelvic pain or pain in the groin may indicate sacral involvement. Pain, itch or discomfort in the eyes, photophobia, or any visual changes might suggest ocular complications. Skin rash, either generalized or affecting the penis or the soles of the feet, might have been noted. The absence of extra-articular symptoms is relatively common and does not exclude a diagnosis of SARA.
Ask about the nature of his recent urethral discharge: was it treated?
Check last sexual contact, other contacts in the last month. Determine gender, origin and location of partners and condom use. Ask about symptoms in a regular partner.
Check past medical history including previous episodes of arthritis, any family history of seronegative arthritis (ankylosing spondylitis, psoriatic arthritis, reactive arthritis). Any recent history of gastroenteritis or trauma may be important.
b) The main differential diagnoses of a monoarthropathy and urethral discharge in a young sexually active man are:
 • gonococcal arthritis
 • other septic arthritis.
There are numerous other possibilities that are much less likely (see Box 5.5). Urethritis is very common in men of this age, so consider the possibility of NGU and an unrelated mechanical knee injury.
c) Factors on examination that may influence your choice of investigation:
 • Systemic symptoms, fever, tachycardia and a tense, hot, monoarthropathy would strongly suggest a septic joint. Systemic symptoms are not a reliable feature of a gonococcal arthritis, which may occur in isolation.

- Pain and stiffness in other joints, tenderness over the sacro-iliac joints, psoriatic rash, conjunctivitis, oral lesions or circinate balanitis suggest a reactive arthritis.

In both cases do a full blood count, ESR, urethral smear for Gram-stain microscopy, gonococcal cultures from the throat, urethra and if he has had sex with men, rectum. Syphilis serology is unlikely to be relevant to the immediate problem but should of course be done, and HIV testing should be offered.

If septic arthritis is suspected, blood cultures and joint aspiration for Gram-stain microscopy and culture may be indicated (neither are likely to be diagnostic in gonococcal arthritis).

If there are any other features of SARA, X-rays of the joint and sacroiliac joints, referral for slit-lamp examination. Testing for HLA B27 is not helpful in diagnosis but may be useful in advising him on the risk of recurrence.

d) Treat him with an antichlamydial antibiotic. Azithromycin 1g stat is first-line therapy, although some clinicians would give an alternative, for example a course of doxycycline because this may be superior in eradicating *U. urealyticum* infection. Supply anti-inflammatory medication (e.g. ibuprofen 400 mg three times daily), advise bed rest, abstinence from sex. Arrange contact tracing and discuss the possible diagnosis and implications. Arrange review fairly soon: in 3 days culture results will be available. One other factor to consider in the absence of any other features of reactive arthritis is whether to treat for possible gonococcal arthritis: Gram-stain microscopy will detect 90% of urethral gonorrhoea, but throat or rectal infection will not be detected. A decision to treat might be based on the clinical picture, his epidemiological risk factors and the local prevalence of gonorrhoea. If infection thought likely, he should be admitted to initiate treatment while awaiting culture results.

Syphilis, herpes simplex virus and other infections causing genital ulceration

6

INTRODUCTION

Infectious causes of ulceration accounted for less than 5% of new diagnoses in GUM clinics in the UK in 1999. In the UK, USA and most parts of the developed world, genital herpes is the most likely of many possible causes of genital ulcer (Box 6.1). In clinics in sub-Saharan Africa and Southeast Asia, more than half of all patients with STI may present

Box 6.1: Causes of genital ulceration	
Infection	Herpes simplex virus 1 Herpes simplex virus 2 Varicella zoster virus
	Primary and secondary syphilis
	Chancroid Lymphogranuloma venereum Granuloma inguinale Pyogenic ulcer Candidiasis (balanitis or vulvitis) Bacterial vaginosis Trichomoniasis TB Scabies
Systemic illness	Crohn's disease Ulcerative colitis
Dermatological conditions (see Ch. 7)	**Local** Plasma cell balanitis Squamous cell carcinoma Genital apthosis Lichen sclerosus/Balanitis xerotica obliterans
	Systemic Behçet's syndrome Stevens-Johnson syndrome
Miscellaneous	Trauma Local allergic reaction (topical creams, *Candida*) Fixed drug eruption

with genital ulceration and chancroid is the commonest diagnosis, sometimes presenting with co-infection with syphilis and/or herpes simplex virus. Lymphogranuloma venereum (LGV) and Donovanosis cause a minority of cases of genital ulceration even in places where the infections are endemic. Other STIs and non-sexually transmitted infections may also be associated with ulceration (Box 6.1). Non-sexually transmitted causes of ulceration are common and include pyogenic ulcers, systemic and local dermatological conditions, reactions to topical and systemic drugs and trauma.

The clinical diagnosis of genital ulceration is notoriously unreliable; atypical herpetic ulcers are common (Fig. 6.1) and primary syphilis (Fig. 6.2) can take almost any form, the clinical picture of both infections being further complicated in people with HIV. In practice in the UK, as other infectious causes of ulceration are comparatively rare (Fig. 6.3), a clinical diagnosis of herpes based on symptoms and signs is likely to be

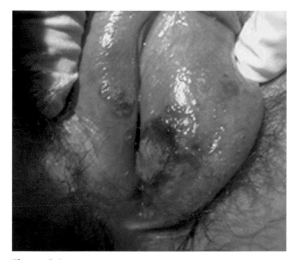

Figure 6.1
Atypical herpetic ulceration of the vulva with haemorrhage

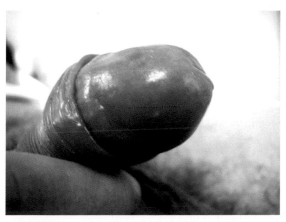

Figure 6.2
Early primary chancre

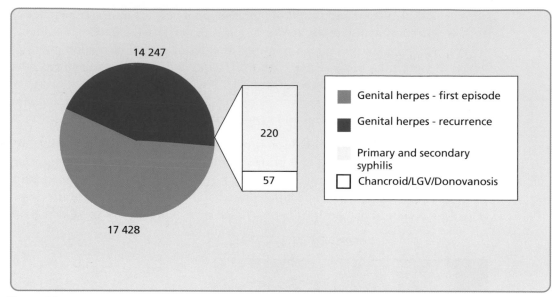

Figure 6.3
Cases of infections causing genital ulceration, UK GUM clinics, 1999
(Data from PHLS, DHSS & PS and the Scottish ISD(D)5 Collaborative Group, 2002.)

correct, but the possibility of other pathology, including syphilis, should be considered in *every* case. The maxim 'any anogenital ulcer is syphilitic or herpetic until proven otherwise' is useful. Painless genital ulcers are only one of many presenting features of primary and secondary syphilis and the diagnosis may be missed at this stage in places where the infection is uncommon. Hence syphilis serology should be routinely performed in all cases of genital ulceration and repeated 90 days later in any case where no other diagnosis is confirmed.

MANAGEMENT OF GENITAL ULCERATION AND SUSPECTED SYPHILIS

HISTORY

Follow the approach described in Chapter 1. Pay particular attention to the nature and development of ulcer(s) and any preceding and accompanying symptoms:

- Solitary or multiple ulcers, pain, timing relative to last sexual contact (incubation period)
- Prodromal symptoms, itch
- Oral ulceration
- Lymph node enlargement, with or without pain
- Accompanying symptoms: rash, fever, joint pain, malaise

- Systemic features
- Previous episodes of ulceration.

Take a detailed history of recent travel and the origin of recent sexual partners to identify cases where tropical infections should be considered. A comprehensive partner history is also useful if contact tracing proves necessary. Ask about symptoms, including ulcers, rash and orolabial herpes (cold sores), in a sexual partner. Recent medication, both oral and topical is important because drug reactions are included in the differential diagnosis. In those with suspected syphilis (because of contact with an infected patient, or positive syphilis serology) inquire also about:

- past history of syphilitic lesions (see below)
- history of yaws or pinta
- previous treatment with penicillins, either for syphilis treatment or for other infections
- history of miscarriage or stillbirth in women
- blood samples taken in the past (may help determine when infected and assist with contact tracing).

Clinical notes: history taking in genital ulceration

- Nature of ulceration
- Painful or painless ulcers
- Timing relative to last sexual contact
- Accompanying symptoms
- Systemic illness
- Partner history
- Travel

EXAMINATION

Check oral cavity, looking for ulcers on the buccal mucosa, palate and tonsils. Examine the skin including the palms and soles for rash. When examining an ulcer consider the appearance of the lesions:

- Single or multiple
- Erosion (epidermis only) or ulcer (dermis exposed)
- The ulcer edge and base
- Presence of slough or bleeding
- Induration (firm or hard to palpation)
- Surrounding oedema.

Note the presence of a urethral or vaginal discharge. Palpate the inguinal lymph nodes, noting the extent of any enlargement, the consistency and any tenderness. The cervical and axillary lymph nodes should also be examined (considering secondary syphilis, co-existing HIV infection). In cases of positive treponemal serology check for the 'tissue paper' scars of old yaws in those from endemic areas.

INVESTIGATION

Full investigation, including dark-ground microscopy, is optimal in every case of genital ulcer. In some settings, such as general practice, this is not possible. In cases of multiple painful ulcer presenting in the UK, the following routine investigations can be used:

1. Swab from ulcer/erosion for detection of HSV. Use a cotton wool-tipped swab, or the swab provided with a commercial testing kit to obtain material from the base of the ulcer. Firm pressure is required to obtain a satisfactory sample. This is painful for the patient who should be prepared for the procedure. If blisters or crusted lesions are present without open ulcers the surface may be broken, with the patient's consent, to obtain a satisfactory sample. The swab is placed into viral transport medium (Hanks) or a commercial kit media.
2. Syphilis serology according to local availability, such as EIA for anti-treponemal IgG, or venereal diseases research laboratory and rapid plasma reagin (VDRL/RPR) tests with *Treponema pallidum* haemagglutination assay (TPHA) (see below).
3. Tests for gonorrhoea, chlamydial infection, trichomoniasis and HIV and hepatitis serology if indicated. If speculum examination is tolerated and discharge is present, tests for bacterial vaginosis and *Candida* (see Ch. 3).
4. Serum sample for storage (to be used at a later date with a convalescent sample for complement fixation tests (CFT) or for type-specific herpes serology if tests for virus identification are unsuccessful).

Using this approach, other causes of ulceration are unlikely to be missed provided:

- routine syphilis serology is always performed
- tests for early syphilis (dark-ground microscopy (DGM) and/or PCR where available) are taken in all cases of solitary or atypical ulcers
- patients with risk factors for topical infection are identified
- follow-up for repeat syphilis serology at 90 days or sooner is ensured.

The diagnosis and further investigation of genital ulceration is shown in Figure 6.4.

In female patients with extensive, painful, initial episode clinical genital herpes, confine examination to the external genitalia, taking a superficial sample for herpes virus identification and serum to store and for syphilis serology. Speculum examination and tests for gonorrhoea, chlamydial infection and trichomoniasis can be taken at a review appointment once the lesions have healed.

Checklist: investigation of painful ulcers

- Swab for herpes simplex identification
- Microscopy for bacterial vaginosis and candidiasis in women
- Syphilis serology
- Serum to store

(plus routine tests for gonorrhoea, chlamydial infection, trichomoniasis)

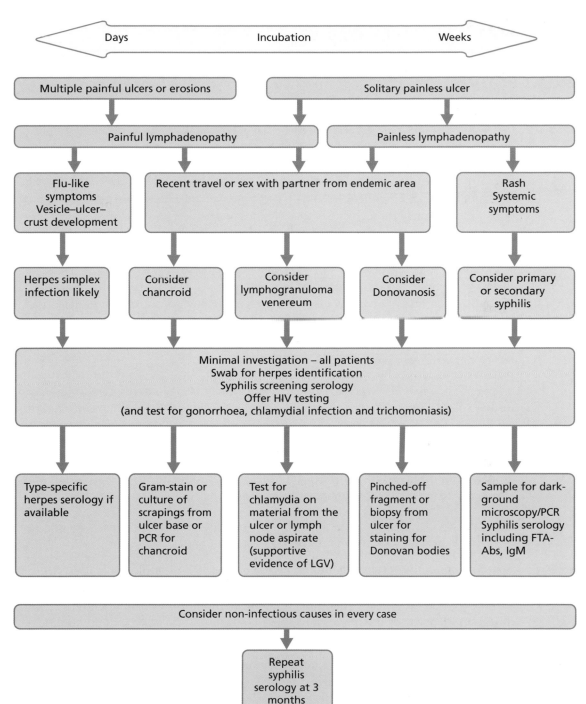

Figure 6.4
Diagnosis of infectious genital ulceration

SYPHILIS

BACKGROUND

The bacterium *Treponema pallidum* was identified as the cause of syphilis in 1905. In the UK, the majority of reported cases of syphilis are diagnosed on serological testing, usually in asymptomatic patients. An upturn in rates in the USA in 2001 after a decade of decline and a dramatic increase in cases in the UK from 1998 has been attributed mainly to outbreaks in homosexual men. In 2002, 1232 cases of primary and secondary syphilis were reported in England, Wales and Northern Ireland. *Treponema pallidum* subspecies *pallidum* can be transmitted sexually through exposure to lesions on the skin and mucous membranes for the first 2–4 years after infection. Infection in the first 2 years after acquisition is classified as early syphilis. Patients presenting during this early infectious stage of the disease may have clinical signs at the site of inoculation, with or without symptoms, described as primary syphilis. Weeks or months later the systemic signs and symptoms of secondary syphilis appear, the most common being rash, mucous membrane lesions and lymphadenopathy. If undiagnosed, clinical signs resolve and, although there is serological evidence of untreated infection, there is no clinical disease. This state is described as early latent syphilis and a recurrence of mucous patches or other signs of secondary syphilis appear in about 25% of cases, rendering the patient highly infectious once more. From 2 years after infection (1 year in the USA), the disease is known as late syphilis. Untreated late syphilis remains asymptomatic and leads to no further complications in 60% of patients. Asymptomatic patients with no clinical evidence of cardiovascular, neurological, or other complications are described as having late latent syphilis. In 30% of untreated patients, gumma of the skin or bone, or cardiovascular or nervous system disease develops between 2 and 30 years after primary infection and is described as tertiary syphilis (Fig. 6.5). Vertical transmission from mother to foetus may occur at any stage, although rarely occurs in pregnancies more than 8 years after initial infection.

PATHOGENESIS AND CLINICAL PRACTICE

Treponema pallidum subsp. *pallidum* is one of several treponemes infecting man. Many are harmless commensals of the mouth, so dark-ground microscopy (see below) of oral lesions is not useful for the diagnosis of syphilis. Non-syphilis treponemes may also contaminate ulcers at other sites and syphilis diagnosed on dark-ground microscopy findings should always be confirmed by serology.

The treponemes vary in both their infectivity and ability to cause disease: *Treponema pallidum* subsp. *pallidum*, the cause of venereal syphilis, is the most infectious and pathogenic: an estimated 50% of contacts are infected. Other subspecies are non-sexually transmitted and cause the diseases yaws, pinta and bejel (Box 6.2). Serological tests for syphilis are unable to distinguish between these treponemal diseases. Pathogenic treponemes are not easily cultured.

Serological testing for syphilis may not prove positive for a week after the appearance of a primary chancre. Direct tests and repeat serology are of vital importance in detecting early syphilis in people presenting with genital ulceration.

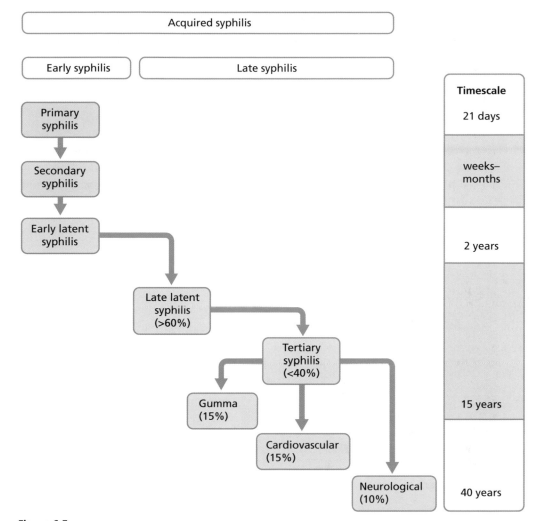

Figure 6.5
Classification and natural history of untreated syphilis

Box 6.2: Non-syphilitic treponemes

Organism	Disease	Region	Clinical manifestations
Treponema pallidum pertenue	yaws	W. Africa, Indonesia, S. America	Cutaneous, bone
Treponema pallidum endemicum	bejel	Middle East, Southern Sahara	As syphilis
Treponema carateum	pinta	South America	Cutaneous only

There is still considerable doubt over whether treponemes are fully eradicated in syphilis therapy. Patients with long-term clinical cure of syphilis may have persistent treponemes in lymph nodes and CNS. This is of particular concern in patients with HIV infection.

CLINICAL FEATURES

Primary syphilis

The chancre, a painless, usually solitary ulcer, appears 9–90 days after sexual contact at the site of initial infection. As the ulcer is sometimes asymptomatic, it may be unnoticed by the patient. Chancres are seen at sites of sexual contact, usually on the genitals: in 99% of heterosexual men, the chancre is on the penis (Fig. 6.6). Any part of the vulva, vagina or cervix may be involved in women (Fig. 6.7). In 30–40% of homosexual men,

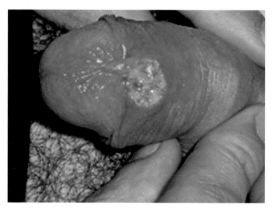

Figure 6.6
Primary chancre of penis

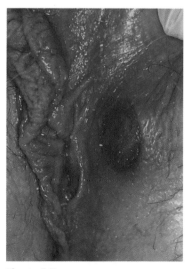

Figure 6.7
Primary chancre of the vulva

and occasionally in women, anorectal chancres are seen. Chancres affecting the fingers and other parts of the skin surface are rare. The early chancre is a firm, dark red macule which ulcerates, enlarging slowly then healing over several weeks. The ulcer is well demarcated, round and clean. It may be indurated and covered with a crust. Serous fluid may appear if firm pressure is applied. The draining lymph nodes are enlarged in 50% of patients but usually painless.

Secondary syphilis

Around 90% of patients with secondary syphilis have a rash (Fig. 6.8). This is usually described as macular or maculopapular, but less commonly pustular, circinate, psoriasiform or other atypical presentations are seen. The rash is generalized, the trunk being affected in 80% and the palms and soles in around half of cases (Fig. 6.9). Up to 75% also have lymphadenopathy. Oral and genital mucous patches (Fig. 6.10), described as snail-track ulcers and condylomata lata are less common, although patients presenting with secondary syphilis often give a history of chancre, or have a persisting chancre. Rare features include hepatitis, optic neuritis, arthritis and peripheral neuropathy.

Early latent syphilis

Early latent syphilis is characterized by positive serological tests for syphilis with a history of symptoms suggestive of infection or a positive syphilis contact in the last 2 years.

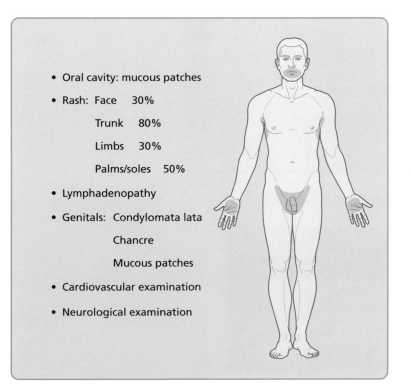

- Oral cavity: mucous patches
- Rash: Face   30%
         Trunk   80%
         Limbs   30%
         Palms/soles   50%
- Lymphadenopathy
- Genitals: Condylomata lata
              Chancre
              Mucous patches
- Cardiovascular examination
- Neurological examination

Examination Box 6.1: Suspected syphilis

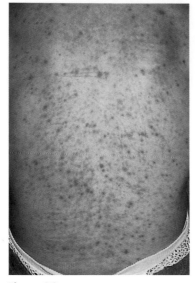

Figure 6.8
Maculopapular rash of secondary syphilis

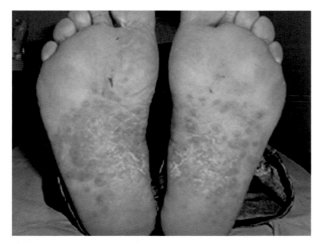

Figure 6.9
Secondary syphilis affecting the soles of the feet

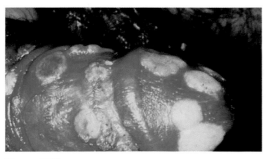

Figure 6.10
Condylomata lata

Late latent syphilis

Positive serological test for syphilis with no history of symptoms or contacts in the last 2 years.

Tertiary syphilis

The gumma, a granuloma resulting from the endarteritis in late syphilis may affect the skin and bones. Cardiovascular syphilis manifests as aortitis and aortic aneurysm. Tabes dorsalis and general paralysis of the insane are the neurological syndromes associated with tertiary syphilis. These conditions are rare and their investigation and management are not covered here.

INVESTIGATION

All patients should undergo screening for STIs. The recent epidemiology of syphilis in the UK and the significance of co-existing HIV infection in syphilis management (Box 6.3) make an HIV test mandatory. A chest X-ray should be taken in latent syphilis and patients with neurological signs should have lumbar puncture to exclude neurosyphilis. Some experts recommend that all patients with HIV co-infection should undergo lumbar puncture but this is not universal practice.

DIAGNOSIS

Most cases of syphilis are detected on serological testing. In the early stages of primary syphilis serological tests may be negative, so tests for the detection of *Treponema pallidum* are used.

Tests for the detection of Treponema pallidum

Dark-ground microscopy

Dark-ground microscopy (DGM) is the only widely available test for demonstration of *Treponema pallidum* in the diagnosis of early syphilis. Clean the chancre with saline and either squeeze the chancre or scrape the surface with gauze, a blade or microscope slide and wait for clotting to begin. Smear a sample of the serum obtained onto a microscope slide or cover slip and examine under the oil immersion lens for the characteristic movements of *Treponema pallidum*. The reliability of the method depends upon experience, and should be taught by an expert microscopist (Fig. 6.11).

Box 6.3: Syphilis and HIV co-infection

Epidemiology	Syphilis strongly associated with increased risk of HIV transmission
	Simultaneous diagnosis of HIV and syphilis not uncommon
Clinical presentation	Atypical rashes
	Meningitis and meningovascular syphilis more common
Diagnosis	Serological response delayed (rare)
	Prozone phenomenon more common
Treatment	Early syphilis: as for non-HIV infected patients
	Late syphilis: treat as neurosyphilis, consider CSF examination

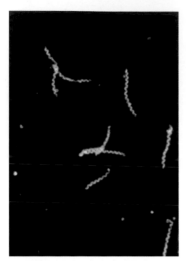

Figure 6.11
Treponema pallidum identified by dark ground microscopy

Direct fluorescent antibody (DFA)

A fluorescein labelled monoclonal antibody to syphilis antigens is applied to an acetone fixed specimen obtained as for dark field microscopy. The test is highly sensitive and specific but not widely available.

Polymerase chain reaction

Although there is currently relatively limited evidence on polymerase chain reaction (PCR) for syphilis diagnosis, the use of the test is likely to increase. PCR for *Treponema pallidum* is comparable to DFA in sensitivity and specificity. It has been used successfully on samples from chancres, lesions of secondary and tertiary syphilis, and in the diagnosis of neurosyphilis.

Serological tests

Serological tests for syphilis include tests for antibodies (IgG, IgM or both) to treponemal antigens and cardiolipin antigens, produced in response to infection (Box 6.4). Antibodies to treponemal antigens are specific to syphilis, but cardiolipin antigen is shared by human (and other mammalian) mitochondria and pathogenic treponemes. Positive tests for antibody to cardiolipin are not exclusively associated with treponemal infection and biological false-positive reactions occur in a number of acute infections, chronic illnesses and other conditions as well as in a few healthy individuals. False-negative results may occur due to a prozone phenomenon, when the level of serum antigen is so high that all available antibody is bound, leaving none to react in the tests. Cardiolipin antigen tests may be used for screening, with tests for treponemal antigen as confirmation of infection. Both types of antigen test can be used to monitor the course of disease and treatment, as the intensity of reaction usually decreases in late disease or after therapy.

Cardiolipin tests include the venereal diseases research laboratory (VDRL) and rapid plasma reagin (RPR) tests. Specific tests for treponemal antigens including enzyme

Box 6.4: Serological tests for syphilis

	Method	Application
Treponemal antigen tests		
Enzyme immunoassay (EIA)	Patient antibodies bind to antigen on microtitre plate Enzyme-labelled anti-immunoglobulin added Automated	Sensitive specific screening test Objectively read (spectrophotometry). Positive from primary infection onward
IgM-EIA	Anti-IgM bound to plate binds IgM in sample. Enzyme-labelled treponemal antigen added	Improves detection of early primary infection
FTA-abs	Indirect immunofluorescence read manually	Standard confirmatory test Subjective
TPHA/TPPA	Erythrocytes (TPHA) or gelatin (TPPA) coated with treponemal antigen agglutinated by patient antibody	Standard recommended screening test in combination with VDRL/RPR Confirmatory test with EIA
Cardiolipin antigen tests		
VDRL slide tests	Agglutination of antigen–antibody complexes read microscopically	Former screening test
VDRL/RPR carbon antigen tests	Agglutination of carbon bound antigen with antibody read by naked eye	Widely used screening test Immediate result

immunoassay to antitreponemal IgG (IgG EIA), enzyme immunoassay to antitreponemal IgM (IgM EIA) and *Treponema pallidum* haemagglutination assay (TPHA). Screening of routine samples may involve VDRL/RPR and TPHA used together, or in many modern laboratories, EIA alone. Positive samples are usually subjected to one or more confirmatory tests.

VDRL/RPR usually fall to low titres in late latent infection and become negative 1 year after treatment of early infection. TPHA usually remains positive for life, even after treatment. Don't expect to make a definitive diagnosis of the stage or treatment status of a patient from serology alone. A comprehensive history and examination is required to assist interpretation (Box 6.5).

TREATMENT

Penicillins are the treatment of choice for all stages of syphilis, on the grounds that there is more accumulated evidence for their long-term effectiveness. Confidence in the effectiveness of treatment in eradicating treponemes from the nervous system is greatest for daily intravenous penicillin therapy, reducing progressively for daily intramuscular injections, weekly intramuscular injections and oral therapy in that order. Box 6.6 shows antibiotics used in syphilis treatment, Box 6.7 selected regimes recommended in current guidelines. Antibiotics other than penicillins have been used with success, but there are no comparative trials. Deep intramuscular injections are painful so patients may be reluctant to agree to parenteral treatment, although adherence to parenteral regimes can be good.

Box 6.5: Interpretation of syphilis serology

Stage				Test		
	IgG-EIA	VDRL	TPHA	FTA-Abs	IgM-EIA
Primary	+ve in 85%	+ve in 75% by 3 weeks after infection Titre 8–16	–ve (may be +ve at low titre: 1/80–160, late in primary)	+ve (may be the only +ve test in very early infection)	+ve
Secondary	+ve	+ve at high titre 16–128	+ve rising to 1/5120	+ve	+ve
Early Latent	+ve	+ve at high then reducing titre	+ve up to 1/5120	+ve	+ve or –ve
Late Latent	+ve	–ve in 30% Low titre <32	always +ve Low titre 1/80–640	+ve	–ve
Treated	+ve	–ve	always +ve Low titre 1/80–640	–ve within 3 months of treatment of early, or 12 months of treatment of late	–ve

(Results cannot be interpreted independently of clinical history. For example, in secondary, recently treated and late latent syphilis results of serological tests may be the same.)

Box 6.6: Drugs used in the treatment of syphilis

Procaine penicillin G	Most accumulated evidence Requires daily injection Painful Treatment reactions: procaine psychosis and penicillin hypersensitivity (rare)
Benzathine penicillin	Weekly injection Painful Reports of treatment failure (though almost all after *single-dose* therapy) Treatment reactions
Amoxycillin plus probenecid	Avoids injection Well tolerated
Doxycycline	Contraindicated in pregnancy Useful in penicillin allergy
Azithromycin, ceftriaxone	Reports of successful use Ceftriaxone has good CNS penetration

The choice of treatment may be based on the patient's wishes, the risk of complications, availability of antibiotics, reports of treatment failure and likelihood of adherence for treatment and long-term follow-up. Non-penicillin regimens are acceptable in patients at low risk of complications, for example HIV-negative patients with primary syphilis. The case for the use of parenteral procaine penicillin is strongest in HIV positive patients, in pregnancy or in patients with tertiary syphilis in whom reports of treatment failure are more common. It is recommended that patients are followed up for life if non-penicillin regimens are used. All patients with HIV and syphilis co-infection should have life-long follow-up.

Box 6.7: Treatment of syphilis

Early syphilis	First-line Procaine penicillin 750 mg (750 000U) intramuscularly daily for 10 days[1] or benzathine penicillin 2.4 MU intramuscularly, two doses 1 week apart Second-line Penicillin allergy Doxycycline 200 mg twice daily for 14 days Second-line Patient declines i.m. injection Amoxycillin 500 mg plus probenecid 500 mg four times daily for 14 days
Late syphilis	First-line Procaine penicillin 750 mg (750 000U) intramuscularly daily for 17 days[1] or benzathine penicillin 2.4 MU intramuscularly for 2 weeks (three doses) Second-line Penicillin allergy Doxycycline 200 mg twice daily for 28 days Second-line Patient declines i.m. injection Amoxycillin 500 mg plus probenecid 500 mg four times daily for 28 days
Neurosyphilis, HIV infection	Procaine penicillin 2 g i.m. plus probenecid 500 mg orally once daily for 17 days or benzylpenicillin 400 mg i.v. 4 hourly (2.4 g/day) for 17 days

[1]The recommended dose of procaine penicillin G is 600 mg (600 000U) but the commonly available preparation is more easily prepared and given at this dosage
(Data from Goh, 2002 and French, 2002.)

Treatment reactions

The Jarisch–Herxheimer reaction is an acute reaction that peaks around 8 hours and resolves within a day of treatment of early syphilis. It occurs in around 50% of primary and 90% of secondary syphilis. It is not dangerous unless there is neurological, cardiovascular or ophthalmic involvement, or in pregnancy. Systemic symptoms including myalgia are followed by fever, chills, and rigors, accompanied by a worsening of the lesions of primary and secondary syphilis. Aspirin relieves symptoms in early infection. A similar flare-up of local lesions in the nervous and cardiovascular systems may cause serious complications if vital structures are involved. Inpatient therapy with prednisolone prior to antibiotic treatment is recommended when treating cardiovascular syphilis, neurosyphilis or optic neuritis.

Procaine psychosis, due to intravenous injection of procaine penicillin and penicillin hypersensitivity may also occur. Always have facilities for resuscitation available and ask about previous penicillin reactions before treating patients with parenteral penicillin.

COUNSELLING, INFORMATION AND PARTNER NOTIFICATION

Considerable time and effort in counselling and partner notification is justified to ensure successful treatment and avoid transmission. The advantages of parenteral treatment over oral therapy should be discussed and the need for follow-up stressed. Patients should be warned of the risk of treatment reaction and advised to avoid intercourse until the treatment course is completed.

Partner notification

Primary syphilis: all partners in the last 90 days should be seen and given epidemiological treatment for possible early syphilis.

Secondary and early latent syphilis: all partners in the last 2 years should be seen and syphilis excluded or epidemiological treatment given. If the most recent contact with the index patient was within 3 months, syphilis serology should be repeated to exclude the diagnosis. If there is any doubt about the timing of contacts or likely attendance for follow-up, a dose of intramuscular benzathine penicillin should be given. This will cure most cases of undetected asymptomatic early infection in patients who are lost to follow-up.

Late syphilis: try to trace a previous serum sample for testing to determine the duration of infection. Long-term partners of those diagnosed with late syphilis and children born to women with late syphilis should be tested to exclude the infection. Deciding who to test in a particular case may be complicated and depends on individual factors including the suspected date of infection and the natural history of the disease.

FOLLOW-UP

The response to treatment is monitored by the cardiolipin antigen tests (VDRL/RPR). A fall of 2 dilutions, causing a 4-fold change in titre (e.g. 256 to 64) is regarded as significant. The decline in titre is more rapid at earlier stages of disease, usually becoming negative within 2 years of treatment of early syphilis. A low titre (<16) may persist long-term after treatment of late infection, but a 4-fold or greater increase in titre after treatment signifies re-infection.

Early syphilis

Review at 1 month after treatment to confirm contact tracing. Repeat serology at 3 months, 6 months and 1 year or until cardiolipin antigen negative.

Late syphilis

As above, but serology should be repeated 6 monthly until 'scrofast', that is unchanged on sequential visits. If non-penicillin antibiotics are used, or if the patient has HIV, follow-up is for life. Patients treated for neurosyphilis undergo repeat CSF examination until the cell count is normal.

GENITAL HERPES

INTRODUCTION

Herpes simplex virus type 1 (HSV 1) and herpes simplex virus type 2 (HSV 2) may cause ulcers of the oral and genital mucosa or may be completely asymptomatic (Fig. 6.12). A diagnosis of genital herpes often causes greater distress than other common STIs and a comprehensive knowledge of the natural history of herpes virus infections is useful in counselling patients. Herpes viruses are transmitted by close contact with the mucous membranes or contaminated body fluids of the oral or genital tract of a person who is infected and is shedding virus. The route of infection is usually the mouth in children; the mouth or genital tract (genital herpes) in adults. Less commonly, the eyes, fingers or other skin sites may be infected with virus from another individual or by self-inoculation. Symptoms, when they occur, range from the mildest discomfort in the absence of clinical signs, to severe systemic illness.

Following infection the virus travels along the axonal nerve fibres of sensory nerves to the dorsal root ganglion supplying the affected area, where it remains latent but reactivates with variable frequency. Symptomatic or asymptomatic recurrence may follow at sites innervated by this nerve root, during which the person is infectious (Box 6.10). Symptoms occurring at the time of first infection are usually more severe than in recurrences.

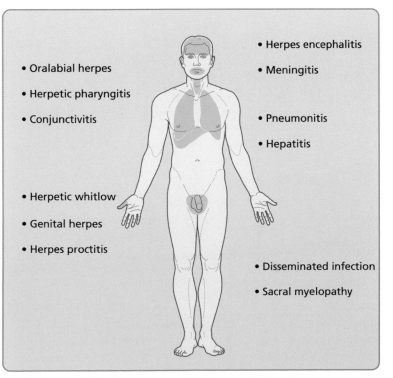

- Oralabial herpes
- Herpetic pharyngitis
- Conjunctivitis

- Herpetic whitlow
- Genital herpes
- Herpes proctitis

- Herpes encephalitis
- Meningitis

- Pneumonitis
- Hepatitis

- Disseminated infection
- Sacral myelopathy

Examination Box 6.2: Diseases caused by herpes simplex virus

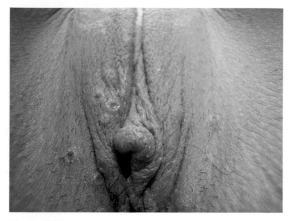

Figure 6.12
Genital herpes: blisters and ulcers

Asymptomatic acquisition followed by a delayed initial symptomatic episode also occurs. Both HSV 1 and HSV 2 may be acquired, and one or both viruses may be carried with or without symptoms. Genital herpes is important because it:

- is common, transmissible, recurrent and incurable
- causes significant physical and psychological morbidity
- causes rare but serious complications in adults and neonates
- is an important cofactor in the transmission of other infections, particularly HIV.

Terminology

Primary infection is an individual's first encounter with a herpes simplex virus (Box 6.8). Primary infection may be with HSV 1 or HSV 2 and may or may not be symptomatic. *Initial episode* genital herpes is the first clinical presentation with genital symptoms of HSV and may be a primary or non-primary infection. About 50% of initial episode genital infections are primary infections. In the UK, HSV 1 and HSV 2 each cause 50% of initial episode genital infections.

Box 6.8: Terminology in genital herpes

Primary infection	An individual's first infection with either herpes virus. May be symptomatic or asymptomatic. Clinically suspected when an initial episode of genital herpes is severe with systemic symptoms. Confirmed only by seroconversion for HSV 1 or 2, or virus detection in a person with previously negative HSV 1 and HSV 2 serology.
Initial episode	First recognised clinical episode of genital herpes. May be a primary infection, a non-primary symptomatic first infection with a new herpes virus (e.g. HSV 2 acquired in an individual already carrying HSV 1), or a delayed symptomatic episode following asymptomatic first infection.
First infection	The first time an individual has acquired a particular herpes virus. If the individual does not already carry a herpes virus this is also the primary infection.

Box 6.9: Seroprevalence of HSV 1 and HSV 2

	Population, prevalence		Associations
HSV 1	Children 1–15, UK general population	25%	Age, gender, ethnic group, social class
	Females 25–30, UK general population	54%	
	Antenatal clinic, London, UK	77%	
HSV 2	UK GUM clinics	15–22%	Lifetime sexual partners, ethnic group,
	UK general population	4–5%	age of first intercourse, history of STD
	USA general population	22%	

NOTES ON EPIDEMIOLOGY

The prevalence of antibodies to HSV 1 in a population depends upon factors including nationality, socioeconomic class and age. HSV 1 is commonly acquired orally in childhood, particularly in poorer socio-economic conditions. Seroprevalence of HSV 1 approaches 100% by middle age in the highest prevalence populations. Sexual behaviour, sexual orientation and gender affect the prevalence of HSV 2. HSV 2 is less prevalent than HSV 1 and is more usually acquired in adulthood and through sexual contact (Box 6.9). The prevalence of HSV 2 in adulthood is increasing and is significantly higher in the USA than in Europe, and in black ethnic groups than in white. The seroprevalence of HSV 2 is 5% in the female general population in the UK, but reaches 80% in African-American women of 60–69 years in the USA. In the past, when acquisition of HSV 1 in childhood was extremely common, the majority of symptomatic initial-episode genital herpes in adults in the UK was due to HSV 2. Age-specific seroprevalence of HSV 1 in childhood has decreased in the UK (e.g. in 10–14 year olds from 34% in 1987 to 24% in 1995). It appears that fewer individuals have now been exposed to HSV by the onset of sexual activity. It is suggested that under these conditions, the first exposure of many individuals to HSV (their primary HSV infection) is by the genital route, often through oro–genital transmission. This suggestion is supported by the finding that over 50% of initial episodes of genital herpes diagnosed in the UK are caused by HSV 1.

PATHOGENESIS AND CLINICAL PRACTICE

Genital herpes due to HSV 1 causes fewer symptomatic recurrences and has a lower rate of viral shedding and onward transmission than HSV 2.

Oral HSV 1 protects against acquiring genital HSV 1. Prior infection with HSV 1 does not appear to affect the likelihood of acquiring HSV 2 or to reduce the frequency of recurrence in HSV 2.

First infection with HSV 2 may have milder symptoms in individuals previously exposed to HSV 1 (i.e. where it is not the primary infection). Those with prior HSV 1 are more likely to have asymptomatic infection with HSV 2. HSV 1 acquisition in someone with prior HSV 2 is rare.

The likelihood of recurrence reduces over time in the majority of cases. The mean decrease in annual recurrence rate is 0.5 per year after primary HSV 1 infection and 0.8 per year after primary HSV 2 infection. However, only one-third of patients have at

141

Box 6.10: Natural history of herpes virus infection

	HSV 1	HSV 2
First infection	63% are symptomatic	37% are symptomatic
Symptomatic recurrence rate	40% of patients in first 6 months after symptomatic primary infection	89% of patients in first 6 months after symptomatic primary infection
	Median rate 0.08 episodes per month (1 per year)	Median rate 0.34 episodes per month (5 per year)
Decline in frequency of symptomatic recurrence	Decrease in annual recurrence rate 0.5 per year	Decrease in annual recurrence rate 0.8 per year
Asymptomatic shedding in the first year after infection (women)	10% of women with primary HSV 1	8% of women with primary HSV 2 23% of women with non-primary HSV 2
Estimates of transmission rate per year to regular sexual partner	Male to female: 1–3% Female to male: 2%	Male to female: 2–17% Female to male: 1–4%

least two fewer recurrences in year 2 than year 1. The median recurrence rate for HSV 2 in year 5 is two per year fewer than in year 1, although 25% of patients have more recurrences in year 5 than year 1.

Men are more likely to have asymptomatic carriage of HSV 2. This may explain why women are more likely to acquire HSV 2 over time.

Asymptomatic viral shedding appears to be about twice as common in HSV 2 as HSV 1, and occurs for longer periods in women.

CLINICAL FEATURES

Sixty-three per cent of HSV 2 and 37% of HSV 1 first infections are asymptomatic. Symptomatic first infections (when an initial episode occurs at the time of first infection) vary in severity and the diagnosis is very commonly missed. Symptoms typically appear between 3 and 9 days after infection, although asymptomatic infection followed by a delayed symptomatic episode within the first year after diagnosis has been observed in around 15% of cases of HSV 2. Initial episodes that are also primary infections are likely to be more severe. HSV 1 or HSV 2 infections are not distinguishable on clinical grounds. Recurrent episodes are similar but are usually confined to the genitals and rarely involve systemic symptoms.

Symptoms

- Pain and dysuria (particularly in women)
- Itching
- Urethral or vaginal discharge
- Systemic symptoms (malaise, fever, myalgia and headache – not usually in recurrent episodes)
- Painful lymphadenopathy affecting the inguinal nodes
- Rectal pain, discharge and tenesmus if lesions affect the rectum.

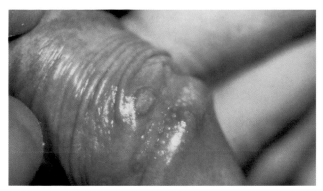

Figure 6.13
Herpetic ulcers of the glans and foreskin

Systemic symptoms tend to peak at 4 days and pain at 10 days after the start of the illness. Some patients experience a prodrome prior to recurrence, such as abnormal sensation in the dermatome supplied by the affected dorsal root ganglion.

Signs

- Erythema, vesicles, pustules, multiple shallow ulcers (Fig. 6.13) or erosions or crusting lesions depending on the stage of infection
- Ulcers may be clean or sloughy and become confluent in severe episodes (Figs 6.14, 6.16)
- Tender inguinal lymphadenopathy in 50%
- Pharyngitis (in primary infection)
- Cervicitis (70–90% in initial episode) (Fig. 6.15)
- Extragenital blisters in 5–6% (Fig. 6.14).

Complications (usually occur in initial episode only)

- Aseptic meningitis
- Transverse myelitis
- Sacral neuropathy (causing urinary retention and constipation)

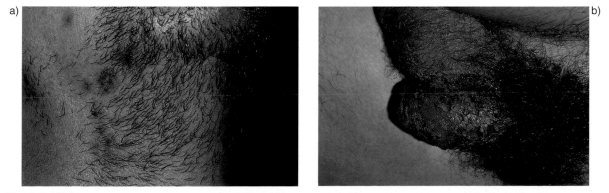

Figure 6.14a,b
Severe primary episode of HSV of the penis with lesions in the beard area – probably autoinoculation

143

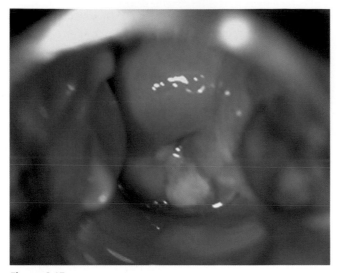

Figure 6.15
Primary herpes affecting the cervix

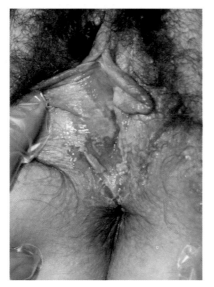

Figure 6.16
Herpetic ulceration of the perineum

- Disseminated infection
- Local extension.

DIAGNOSIS

The significant psychological impact of herpes on the patient may be heightened by uncertainty, so it's important to confirm the diagnosis. This may not be possible, particularly with culture-based tests and in late or recurrent episodes. Identifying the virus type can also be useful in counselling patients regarding prognosis. Tests for virus detection and for herpes antibody are available and in any initial episode, samples for virus identification and serum for serological testing should be taken.

Virus detection

Culture of the virus in an immortal cell culture line is sensitive only in the vesicular and pustular stages of infection. It allows viral typing and is widely used but is labour intensive. Antigen detection methods are cheap and some allow near-patient testing, but sensitivity is low and viral typing is not possible. PCR is increasingly used, allows viral typing and is more sensitive than cell culture.

Serological tests

Complement fixation tests (CFT) for herpes antibody are not type-specific and are now rarely used. They require a baseline and convalescent sample and will detect only primary infection. Type-specific serological tests identify type specific antigens by Western blot or antibodies to glycoprotein gG-1 and gG-2 to confirm past infection with HSV 1 and HSV 2 respectively. Glycoprotein g assays are 81–100% sensitive and 97–100% specific. They have made a major contribution to recent understanding of the epidemiology and natural history of herpes virus infection. They are usually positive within 8 weeks of first infection. Their role in diagnosis and in providing information to support patient counselling is subject to debate. A major concern is the risk of false-positive results in low prevalence populations. Potential uses and some of the factors under debate are outlined in Box 6.11.

MANAGEMENT OF GENITAL HERPES

The patient may be faced with adjusting to a stigmatized, incurable, chronic condition while feeling physically unwell, viraemic and in severe discomfort. Management involves

---

Box 6.11: Use of type-specific serological tests in genital herpes

Indication	Benefits	Risks
Identification of women at risk of HSV infection in late pregnancy by testing the woman and her partner	Potential to avert first infection at term and risk of neonatal herpes in serodiscordant couples	No intervention proven to avoid transmission Neonatal herpes is rare Not cost-effective
Assessment of patients with history of possible herpes but no lesions at presentation, undiagnosed genital ulceration	Avoids repeated attempts to diagnose by viral detection	Positive serology doesn't confirm symptoms are due to HSV
Assessment of first episode genital herpes in a regular relationship	Identify delayed initial episode (if seropositive at presentation) Identify asymptomatic partner as source of infection	Both partners must be tested Risk of false positive
Patients with current or previous sexual partners with genital herpes	Informed decision on future risk, avoidance of transmission	Limited ability to avoid transmission through abstinence/condoms Risk of false positive

practical, symptomatic and emotional support, and can usually be done as an outpatient. Admission is indicated in first episode infection complicated by:

- pregnancy
- immunosuppression
- disseminated infection
- symptoms of meningism
- urinary retention
- inability to self-care.

Physical symptoms

Start antiviral therapy immediately in clinically diagnosed initial episodes. Salt baths give relief and topical soft paraffin eases discomfort. Regular systemic analgesia (e.g. ibuprofen) helps with local pain and systemic symptoms. Local analgesics such as lignocaine gel are useful for severe cases and as a last resort to avoid catheterization. Pain is often worse when urinating, so advise to urinate in the bath, or with a shower spray directed onto the genitals.

Other practical measures

Maintain fluid intake, rest and take time off work if possible. Patients may fear disclosure of the diagnosis, so offer an alternative explanation, a 'sick note' or brief letter with a non-specific diagnosis for the patient to use. In patients with urinary retention, or who are becoming dehydrated due to fluid restriction, catheterization is occasionally indicated. Supra pubic catheterization is recommended, although there is no hard evidence to support its superiority over a urethral catheter.

Antiviral drugs

The drugs available are aciclovir, valaciclovir and famciclovir. Treatment reduces the duration of symptoms and of viral shedding and reduces the time to healing in initial and recurrent episodes. There is no substantial evidence of the superiority of one drug over another in terms of clinical effectiveness, so choice is based on cost, availability and dosage convenience. Oral treatment is usually given, although intravenous aciclovir may be used in serious or disseminated infection, or in the immunosuppressed. Topical aciclovir cream is only occasionally useful in the treatment of recurrences.

Treatment of genital herpes with antiviral drugs (Boxes 6.12, 6.13) is indicated in:

- initial episode primary and non-primary infection. Treatment should be given on clinical diagnosis if lesions are less than 5 days old, if new lesions are appearing or in any severe episode with evidence of active lesions.
- recurrent episodes. Treatment of recurrences with self-initiated therapy can also be used, but is effective only if started during the prodrome or the first 24 hours of lesions developing and shortens the duration of symptoms and viral shedding by a median of 1–2 days. Even so, some patients find this very helpful. In a minority of cases, treatment started in the prodrome may avert the episode.

Box 6.12: Treatment of genital herpes[1]

Initial episode[2,3]	Valaciclovir 500 mg twice daily for 5 to 10 days or aciclovir 200 mg five times a day for 5 to 10 days[3]
Recurrent episode (intermittent treatment)[3]	Aciclovir 200 mg five times a day for 5 days or valaciclovir 500 mg twice daily for 3 days
Frequent recurrences (suppressive therapy)[3]	First-line Aciclovir 400 mg twice daily or valaciclovir 500 mg once daily If recurrences not suppressed: second-line Aciclovir 200 mg four times daily or valaciclovir 250 mg twice daily

[1]Evidence level 1b for all treatments
[2]There is no evidence that 10 days' therapy is superior to 5 in initial episode GH. CDC guidelines recommend the longer course and some experts recommend the use of up to 14 days' therapy in initial episode GH. One option is to review on the fifth day to confirm that lesions are resolving and continue therapy only in severe cases. Studies comparing the use of aciclovir, valaciclovir and famciclovir have shown equivalence in the treatment of initial and recurrent episode GH and suppression. Famciclovir is not included here only because of its higher cost.
[3]Other dosage/frequency combinations have been shown to be effective
(Data from Herpes Simplex Advisory Panel, 2001.)

Box 6.13: Drugs used in the treatment of herpes infections

	Advantages	Disadvantages
Aciclovir	Greatest accumulated safety data for long-term use Intravenous form for serious infection Inexpensive generic available	Frequent dosage Low oral bioavailability
Valaciclovir	Infrequent dosage (good oral bioavailability – equivalent to IV aciclovir) Effectiveness comparable to aciclovir	Expensive
Famciclovir	Infrequent dosage Affects natural history of disease in mice – effect in humans unknown	Very expensive Less accumulated evidence

- frequent recurrences. Suppressive therapy is given if recurrences are severe, frequent or cause psychological distress. Aciclovir prevents recurrences in around 75% of people taking it continuously. It also reduces the frequency of subclinical viral shedding, which will, in theory, reduce the chance of transmission. There is no evidence of adverse effect of continuous aciclovir therapy for several years.

It's important that the patient is aware that treatment of an acute initial or recurrent episode won't affect the future course of the disease and suppressive therapy won't affect the natural history of the disease once it is discontinued.

Box 6.14: Patient information in genital herpes

Patient concern	Points to discuss
Sequelae (does it lead to anything else?)	No. HSV may be a cofactor in, but not the cause of, cervical cancer
Transmission to partners (see Box 6.10)	Risk highest when symptomatic, so abstain during recurrence May occur when asymptomatic Risk with HSV 2 > HSV 1 Reduced by condom use (evidence for male–female only) Initial episode occurring years into monogamous long-term relationship is likely to be primary infection. Partner likely to be already infected Type specific serology may be useful in determining if partner infected in some cases
Pregnancy	No effect on fertility Risk of transmission from recurrence in pregnancy is low
Telling partners	Advise to tell current and potential partners Support with when and how to tell
Recurrences	Very variable natural history (see Box 6.10) Recurrences more likely in the first year Treatment may reduce severity and duration but not necessary if mild
Anger towards partner	Common infection. Often asymptomatic Partner likely to be unaware of infection Most people acquire virus from someone without symptoms
Fears regarding infidelity in a regular relationship	Low rate of partner-to-partner transmission in regular relationship – so transmission may occur after long period of monogamy Possibility of oro-genital transmission
Partners are mutual first sexual partners	Possibility of oro-genital transmission

PATIENT INFORMATION, COUNSELLING AND SUPPORT

The emotional reaction to herpes may be severe. Patients may experience distress, depression, fear of rejection, loss of self-esteem and psychosexual problems. Concern about current and future relationships, pregnancy and fertility are common. Patient support groups are particularly helpful and provide high-quality information. The information given should be tailored to the patient's personal circumstances, concerns and the type of herpes virus. A balance is required between preventing onward transmission of the virus by modifying behaviour, for which the evidence is limited, and minimizing the psychological impact of the disease. Some of the concerns that may arise are outlined in Box 6.14.

OTHER INFECTIVE CAUSES OF GENITAL ULCERATION

Other infective causes of ulceration are rare in developed nations where they are seen almost exclusively in those who have visited the tropics. See Further reading for recent reviews of tropical infections.

CHANCROID

Chancroid is a rare cause of genital ulceration in the UK (Figs 6.17, 6.18). It is an important cofactor in HIV transmission; co-infection with HIV, herpes and syphilis is not unusual. The incubation period is short (usually less than 7 days) and the multiple, painful ulcers may be similar to herpes but are characteristically ragged edged and undermined. Tender inguinal lymphadenopathy occurs in one-third of cases and the nodes may suppurate. Culture, if available is up to 80% sensitive. PCR may be available in some centres. Treat with azithromycin 1 g orally single dose, or erythromycin 500 mg orally three times a day for 7 days. Treat all contacts within the last 10 days. Do an HIV test at presentation and after 3 months.

LYMPHOGRANULOMA VENEREUM

Lymphogranuloma venereum (LGV) is a chlamydial infection with a short incubation period (3–21 days). The primary lesion, a painless ulcer with undermined edges, appears then heals and is commonly unnoticed. Weeks later, tender inguinal lymphadenopathy develops, with abscess formation (buboes) (Fig. 6.19) and if untreated, scarring, strictures and fistulae. Diagnosis is by culture of C. *trachomatis* or specific serological tests. Doxycycline 100 mg twice daily for three weeks is the treatment of choice.

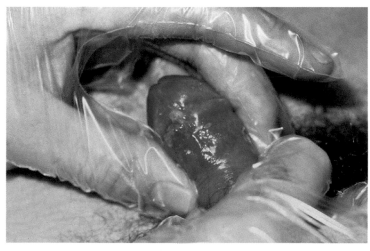

Figure 6.17
Chancroid of penis

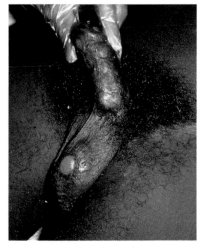

Figure 6.18
Chancroid of the penis with scrotal 'kiss' lesions

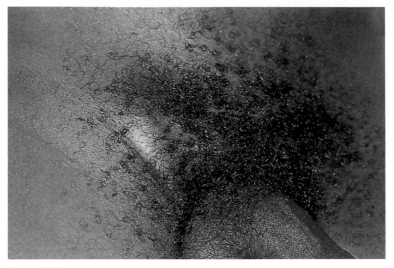

Figure 6.19
Bubo of LGV

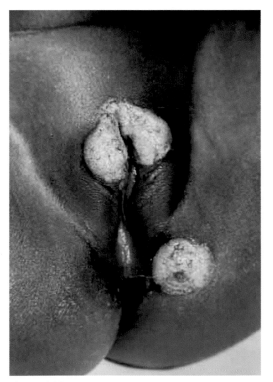

Figure 6.20
Donovanosis

DONOVANOSIS

Donovanosis (Fig. 6.20) is caused by the bacterium *Klebsiella granulomatis*. It causes a slow growing, soft, very erythematous ulcer, usually affecting the anogenital area in socially deprived populations in South Asia and Papua New Guinea. Biopsy material from the base or the edge of the lesion may be Giemsa stained and examined under the microscope to identify the organism. Treatment with doxycycline or ciprofloxacin is effective.

ZOSTER

Zoster affecting a sacral nerve root may present with signs and symptoms indistinguishable from symptomatic genital herpes. The clearly unilateral dermatomal distribution of the lesions gives a clue to the diagnosis. Treatment is with high-dose aciclovir (see Ch. 10, Box 10.2).

Further Reading

Benedetti J, Corey L, Ashley R. Recurrence rates in genital herpes after symptomatic first episode infection. Ann Intern Med 1994; 121: 847-854.

Fenton KA, Nicoll A, Kinghorn G. Resurgence of syphilis in England: time for more radical and nationally coordinated approaches. Sex Transm Infect 2001; 77: 309–310 (and accompanying articles in a Syphilis Symposium).

French P. UK national guidelines on the management of late syphilis. 2002. www.bashh.org/guidelines/late%20$%20final%20b%2031%2012%202002.pdf

Goh B. UK national guidelines on the management of early syphilis. 2002. www.bashh.org/guidelines/early$final0502.pdf

Herpes Simplex Advisory Panel. National guidelines for the management of genital herpes 2001. www.bashh.org/guidelines/hsv%2006%2001.pdf

Langenberg AGM, Corey L, Ashley RL et al. A prospective study of new infections with herpes simplex virus type 1 and type 2. N Engl Jour Med 1999; 341: 1432–1438.

Lewis DA. Chancroid: clinical manifestations, diagnosis and management. Sex Transm Infect 2003; 79: 68-71.

Mindel A, Tovey SJ, Timmins DJ, Williams P. Primary and secondary syphilis, 20 years' experience. 2. Clinical features. Genitourin Med 1989; 65: 1–3.

Munday PE, Vuddamalay J, Slomka MJ, Brown DWG. Role of type specific herpes simplex virus serology in the diagnosis and management of genital herpes. Sex Transm Infect 1998; 74: 175–178.

PHLS, DHSS & PS and the Scottish ISD(D)5 Collaborative Group. Sexually Transmitted Infections in the UK: New episodes seen at genitourinary medicine clinics, 1991–2001. London; Public Health Laboratory Service: 2002.

Scoular A. Using the evidence base on genital herpes: optimising the use of diagnostic tests and information provision. Sex Transm Infect 2002; 78: 160–165.

SELF-ASSESSMENT

Question 1

A 50-year-old man attends your clinic with a single painless ulcer on his glans penis, present for 2 weeks. He last had sex 17 days ago with his wife of 22 years. About a month ago he had receptive and insertive oral sex, without a condom, with a male partner in a sauna.

What is the most important diagnosis to confirm or exclude, and what are the priorities for management on his initial visit?

Question 2

A 17-year-old girl presents with a 5-day history of worsening dysuria, fever, headache and myalgia. She has not passed urine for 18 hours due to the pain. She has had a regular 19-year-old male partner (her first) for 2 years. On examination she has multiple small, sloughy ulcers over the vulva and perineum. The clinical diagnosis is initial episode genital herpes.
a) Briefly outline essential features of assessment and diagnosis.
b) What factors would influence you to admit her to hospital? What advice would you give on self-care at home?
c) At her review appointment 3 weeks later PCR is positive for HSV 1. What information might you give her?
d) What advice and information can you give him?

Answers
1) Primary syphilis
   The main priorities are:
   Diagnosis: do dark-ground microscopy, direct fluorescent antibody test or PCR according to availability and repeat if necessary on 3 consecutive days. Blood for syphilis serology should be taken. Anti-treponemal IgM EIA and FTA-abs should be specifically requested from the laboratory and are likely to be positive if the chancre has been present for a week.
   HIV risk: explore previous risks in relation to HIV infection. Co-existing HIV infection may influence further management. Has he ever had an HIV test? Offer a test. Discuss re-testing after window period.
   Partner notification: detailed discussion about his wife and sauna partners, plus any other contacts in the last 3 months, is appropriate at first visit in case syphilis is diagnosed. Contact tracing in syphilis is given very high priority, particularly where a case is linked to a sex establishment.
   Make certain of follow-up for further testing and/or treatment and of the details of sexual contacts.
2)
a) • Confirm last menstrual period and possibility of pregnancy.
   • Examine for urinary retention, dehydration, oropharyngeal ulceration and evidence of disseminated herpes.
   • Test for herpes virus, herpes and syphilis serology.

b) Evidence of meningism, significant dehydration, inability to swallow medication, urinary retention, or the lack of a carer might necessitate admission. Most patients can be managed as outpatients. Advise to pass urine in the bath, give local analgesic gel, encourage fluid intake, rest until fully recovered. A 10-day course of oral antiviral therapy, though not evidence based, is prudent in a severe initial episode.

c) This is likely to have been primary infection, acquired from her current partner, either from his mouth or his genitals. There is no implication of infidelity – he may not necessarily ever have had another sexual partner. There is a 40% chance of a recurrence in the first 6 months, which would be much less severe than the initial episode. Treatment is not necessary for recurrences unless they are severe or frequent. The chance of passing the virus back to her partner's genitals and causing a symptomatic episode after acquiring it orally is not known, but is low enough to be disregarded.

d) He has either oral or genital HSV 1, or both. It will not be possible to determine the sites of infection unless he has a history of symptoms. More than half the population have this virus during life, so he is not unusual. If he has not already had symptoms of herpes, he is unlikely to get them in future (unless he acquires HSV 2). Advise him on preventing STI transmission to or from future partners through condom use, but be cautious about suggesting that transmission of herpes virus is effectively prevented, as there is little evidence for this. The risk of transmission of HSV 1 if asymptomatic is low.

Infections and other conditions of the genital skin

INTRODUCTION

Conditions of diverse aetiology affect the skin of the external genitalia and consequently present to sexual health clinics. Patients may complain of discomfort, itch or pain, or have concerns that a change in appearance of the genital skin causing no other symptoms is due to a sexually transmitted infection. Both sexually transmitted and non-sexually transmitted skin conditions may have significant psychological impact, affecting body image and precipitating anxiety, sexual dysfunction and relationship problems. Appropriate explanation and reassurance is an important part of management. Genital types of human papilloma virus are almost always sexually transmitted and genital warts are the commonest manifestation of sexually transmissible infection affecting the genital skin. Several other skin infections may be, but are not exclusively transmitted through sexual contact, including the viral infection molluscum contagiosum and the arthropod *Sarcoptes scabiei*. Non-sexually transmitted infections commonly encountered include genital candidiasis, tinea cruris and infective balanitis or balanoposthitis. Non-infective conditions of the genital skin include generalized skin diseases, for example psoriasis, eczema and lichen planus, all of which may affect only the genitals, or present in the genital area prior to appearing in other parts of the body. A number of relatively uncommon conditions confined to the genital skin, including plasma-cell balanitis and lichen sclerosus are not infrequently seen in sexual health clinics. Malignancies and premalignant conditions are seen in the genital area and biopsy is required where the differential diagnosis of a lesion includes this possibility. Biopsy is also useful if the diagnosis cannot be made on clinical grounds and this affects management. Only the most commonplace of the wide range of non-sexually transmitted infections and non-infectious conditions will be covered here. Box 7.1 lists the commoner conditions affecting the genital skin.

CLINICAL ASSESSMENT

Skin conditions presenting in the sexual health setting fall into two broad groups. In most, the presenting symptoms will suggest a diagnosis immediately and examination confirms the diagnosis, for example the majority of newly noticed lumps in young people will be genital warts (Figs 7.1, 7.2). In the rest, the differential diagnosis is often broad and a detailed history and examination is required prior to investigation including biopsy.

Box 7.1: Conditions affecting the genital skin

STIs	Genital warts
	Pediculosis pubis
Other infections	Infective balanitis/balanoposthitis
	Molluscum contagiosum
	Scabies
	Candidiasis
	Tinea
Systemic skin conditions	Eczema/dermatitis
	Psoriasis
	Lichen planus
	Pemphigus
Local skin conditions	Lichen sclerosus
	Lichen simplex
	Plasma cell balanitis
	Erythroplasia of Queyrat
	Circinate balanitis
	Carcinoma
Ulcers	STIs (Ch. 6)
	Fixed drug eruption
	Stevens–Johnson syndrome
	Apthous ulcers
	Behçet's disease

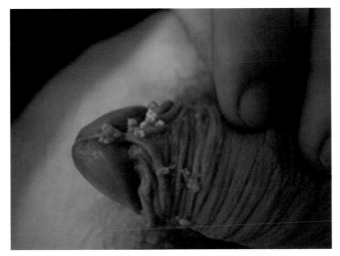

Figure 7.1
Warts on the penis

History

Ask about the timescale and development of changes in the skin, particularly in relation to recent sexual contacts, which may be important if contact tracing is required. Ask about itch, pain, bleeding and other accompanying symptoms that might suggest STI, such as discharge. Explore concerns about possible diagnoses and any impact on current

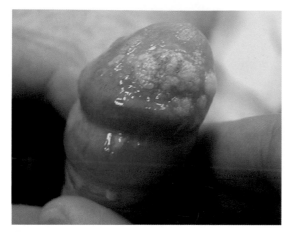

Figure 7.2
Warts on the glans with balanitis

relationship and sex life. There may be a history of similar lesions (warts or molluscum contagiosum) in a partner. Other features that may be relevant include:

- Changes elsewhere in the skin
- Oral lesions
- A personal or family history of skin problems or allergy
- Self-initiated treatments
- Recent oral and topical treatments
- Previous episodes of the same problem.

Patients often diagnose (and misdiagnose) warts themselves. Men, particularly teenagers, with filiform coronal papillae (Fig. 7.3) or prominent sebaceous glands (Fordyce's spots) (see Fig. 1.10) may present as 'warts', having noticed them after sexual activity, or when self-examining because of concern about possible STI.

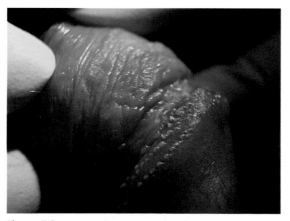

Figure 7.3
Coronal papillae

Examination

Unless the diagnosis is immediately apparent from the clinical history, it is usually appropriate to examine the whole of the skin surface, including the scalp, oral cavity (syphilis, Behçet's, lichen planus), wrists, hands and feet (scabies, lichen planus, psoriasis). When examining a skin lesion in the genitals, the use of a hand lens can be useful. It may, for example, allow you to distinguish the rough, keratinized surface of even very small warts from the umbilicated lesions of molluscum contagiosum. Examine the urethral meatus and perianal area in all cases.

Investigation

Patients presenting with genital warts should always have tests for sexually transmitted infections (up to 30% have another STI). An STI screen should be offered to most other sexually active people and those at low risk who have presented because of concern that symptoms are due to STI. Biopsy should be considered where there is an atypical or pigmented single wart. Lesions that are pigmented, rapidly growing, ulcerate or bleed should also be biopsied. If probable molluscum contagiosum infection needs confirmation, remove 'pearly' core from lesions with the tip of a needle, placing in a dry universal container and sending to virology for electron microscopy for pox virus. Where fungal infection is suspected, skin scrapings from the margin of a lesion may be suspended in 10% potassium hydroxide for microscopy. Skin scraping or hairs can be cultured for *Candida* or tinea infection. If Gram-stain microscopy is to be done to diagnose yeast infection, a piece of double-sided sticky tape attached to a microscope slide and pressed onto the lesion, then onto a glass slide gives a better preparation than a Dacron swab.

In many cases, skin biopsy is useful. It can usually be performed in the clinic without special facilities. The procedure should be explained to the patient and written consent recorded in the case notes. Lignocaine 1–2% with adrenaline is infiltrated into the lesion. A punch biopsy is pressed into the skin, including the whole lesion or a representative sample, and rotated before lifting the biopsy with forceps and releasing the base. A single suture is sufficient to allow healing, but patients should be warned that they are likely to be left with a small scar.

GENITAL WARTS

BACKGROUND

Genital warts are the most frequently diagnosed STI in the developed world and until recently, were the commonest problem presenting to GUM clinics in the UK. They are a cosmetic problem; nevertheless they are disfiguring and often recurrent. Available treatments are not curative. The psychological impact of genital warts and their effect on sexual function and relationships is often disproportionate to their clinical severity. Human papillomavirus (HPV) infections cause substantial morbidity and mortality from genital cancers, but the presence of genital warts is a poor predictor of risk of such anogenital cancer. Concern about the risk of cancer and long-term carriage of HPV may heighten the psychological impact of genital warts and giving appropriately detailed information and reassurance is an important part of management. Figure 7.4 illustrates the number of cases of warts seen in GUM clinics in the UK.

EPIDEMIOLOGY, PATHOGENESIS AND CLINICAL PRACTICE

Although the majority of genital infections with human papillomavirus (HPV) are asymptomatic, approximately 0.2–0.8% of the adult population are diagnosed each year with genital warts. An estimated 20–50% of young sexually active adults have HPV infection and the lifetime risk of being infected with at least one HPV subtype may be as high as 80%.

The majority (90%) of genital warts are caused by HPV subtypes 6 and 11, which are 'low risk' viruses – being implicated in low-grade, but not high-grade squamous intraepithelial lesions (SILs). HPV types 16, 18, 31 and 33 are among those implicated in the development of high-grade SILs and cervical, vulval, vaginal and anal carcinomas (Box 7.2).

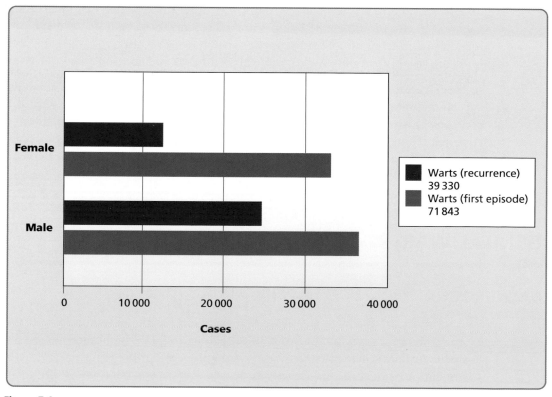

Figure 7.4
First episode and recurrent genital warts, UK GUM clinics 1999
(Data from PHLS, DHSS & PS and the Scottish ISD(D)5 Collaborative Group, 2002.)

6,11	Anogenital warts (condylomata acuminata)
6,11,16,18,31	Squamous intraepithelial lesions of the genitals
16,18,31,	Carcinomas

Genital warts are almost always sexually transmitted, and HPV appears to be highly infectious. Transfer by fomites is thought to be relatively uncommon, but oral– and hand–genital transmission is possible. Warts are usually seen in areas subjected to abrasion during intercourse: minor epithelial damage probably facilitates viral entry.

DIAGNOSIS

The patient usually notices one or more lumps affecting the genitals, perineum or perianal area. Occasionally the warts are unnoticed by the patient but identified at a routine (e.g. cervical smear) examination. Urethral warts may present with urethral discharge, bleeding or disruption of the urinary stream (Fig. 7.5). Mild itch and occasionally pain may accompany warts, particularly in the early stages, but more severe itch, particularly in women, is often due to accompanying candidal infection. The appearance is variable and morphology depends upon site: soft, fleshy, hyperplastic warts (condylomata acuminata) are commonly seen on the moist skin of the glans and subpreputial area in men, on the hymenal remnants or at the introitus in women and at the anal margin in both sexes (Fig. 7.6). Papular, sometimes keratotic, sessile warts are seen on dry skin on the shaft of the penis, on the labia majora and perineum, in the groin or perianally. It is not unusual for concerned patients (especially those with a past history of warts) to present with concerns about very small lesions. A hand lens is useful to distinguish warts from anatomical features such as coronal papillae, vestibular papillae, skin tags or sebaceous glands. It is not usually helpful to treat very minor lesions of unknown aetiology in order

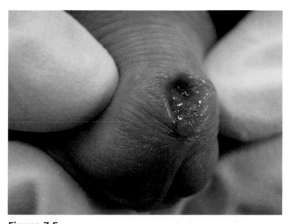

Figure 7.5
Intrameatal warts

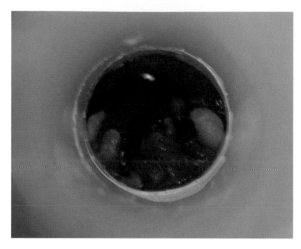

Figure 7.6
Intra-anal warts at proctoscopy

to satisfy hypervigilant patients, who may become even more concerned if the lesion persists. The administration of acetic acid to genital skin to identify subclinical wart virus infection is unreliable and of limited clinical use. The incubation period of warts in one study was 3 weeks to 8 months, average 2.8 months. It is, therefore, usual to see warts present within a year of a new regular relationship. However, warts are seen in patients who appear to give a reliable history of no sexual contact, or contact with one monogamous partner, for several years.

TREATMENT

It should always be clear to the patient (and doctor) that treatment is for cosmetic reasons only. The natural history of genital warts is that infectivity reduces over time, but the evidence that treatment affects this is limited. Where treatment is repeatedly unsuccessful or access is difficult, a balance must be made between the inconvenience of treatment and the possible benefit. The treatments in clinical use include:

- ablation by cautery, freezing, excision, laser or chemical means (Fig. 7.7)
- antimitotic agents such as podophyllotoxin and 5-fluorouracil
- modification of the cellular immune response to wart virus.

Many treatments are available and have been shown to be more effective than placebo in clearing warts or reducing wart area. All treatments have high relapse rates. There are few studies comparing the effect of one treatment modality with another and no one treatment is regarded as superior. There is good evidence that podophyllin solution, for years a mainstay of wart therapy, is less effective than alternatives. Non-comparative trials of imiquimod 5% cream suggest that the relapse rate may be lower than for other treatments. Other than this, there is little to choose between methods. Treatment choice should be made on the grounds of patient preference, convenience and cost. Combinations of treatments (e.g. cryotherapy plus podophyllotoxin) are sometimes prescribed but have been little studied. The number of warts at presentation and the wart

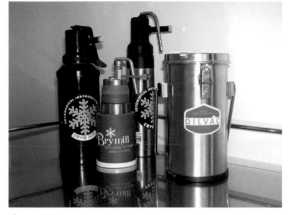

Figure 7.7
Liquid nitrogen cryotherapy equipment

a)

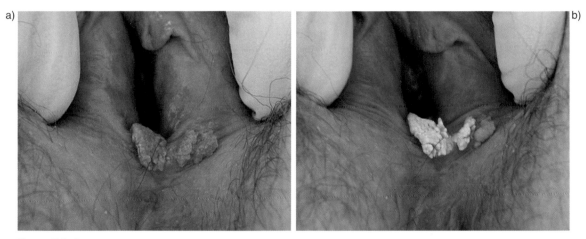

b)

Figure 7.8a,b
Cryotherapy applied to genital warts

area affects the time to clearance, and satisfactory outcome in wart treatment is more likely if treatment is changed when unsuccessful. Introducing protocols for the treatment of genital warts has been shown to improve outcomes. Treatments available for genital warts are shown in Box 7.3. Details on the use of the widely available methods of cryotherapy (Fig. 7.8), podophyllotoxin and imiquimod are given in Box 7.4 and some suggestions on first- and second-line treatments in different situations in Box 7.5. Local treatment protocols will depend upon the skills available, the cost of treatment and the experience of the practitioner – those suggested here are not necessarily any more effective than the alternatives.

PATIENT INFORMATION

- Latent period is months, may be years.
- Asymptomatic carriage is common (>90%).
- There is not necessarily implication of infidelity in a regular relationship.

161

Box 7.3: Advantages and disadvantages of genital wart therapies

	Advantages	Disadvantages
Ablative therapies		
Cryotherapy	Inexpensive equipment Skills easily acquired Good for small numbers of warts Scarring rare	Usually more than one visit Requires trained staff Some pain and occasionally ulceration after treatment Less good for perianal warts
Excision	Good for 1 or 2 warts resistant to other therapies Single-visit therapy Scissor excision is straightforward	Requires time, appropriate equipment and assistance Local anaesthetic required Haemostasis required
Electrocautery	High initial clearance rate	Concerns re risks to staff of vapourised HPV – requires extraction system Local anaesthetic required Risk of scarring
Carbon dioxide laser	Useful if extensive warts, intravaginal or cervical warts, or intraepithelial neoplasia	Expensive equipment Specialist procedure
Trichloroacetic acid	Can be used at most sites Inexpensive Effective for cervical and anal warts	Burning and irritation at treatment site Must be clinic applied Weekly therapy Risk of scarring
Antimitotic agents		
Podophyllin	Inexpensive	Teratogenic Concentrations not standardized Usually applied in clinic Inferior to podophyllotoxin
Podophyllotoxin	Home application Effective	Licensed for use in perianal warts only (not vaginal, urethral or anal) Not used in pregnancy or breast-feeding
5-fluorouracil	Effective for intraurethral and vaginal warts	
Immune-response modifier		
Imiquimod 5% cream	Home application Expensive ? Lower relapse rate Some evidence of cost-effectiveness Licensed for use in perianal warts	Expensive

- Spread is almost always sexual.
- New warts may appear even during treatment.
- Warts may recur, although the probability of recurrence diminishes with time.
- The vast majority of genital warts (>85%) are caused by viruses having no connection with cervical carcinoma.
- Women with genital warts require routine 3 yearly cervical smears only and no additional intervention or screening.

Box 7.4: Use of cryotherapy, podophyllotoxin and imiquimod

Method	Use
Cryotherapy with liquid nitrogen	Can be applied using cotton wool swabs, an insulated flask, or a closed system with a metal 'probe'. In all cases, a 'bloom' of freezing should be maintained around each wart for at least 30 seconds. Tolerability varies from patient to patient. If discomfort experienced supply anaesthetic cream (e.g. EMLA) for application prior to attending the clinic. Repeat treatment at two weekly intervals for 5 cycles
Podophyllotoxin	Podophyllotoxin 0.5% solution (Warticon, Condyline, Podofilox). Podophyllotoxin 0.15% cream or gel (Warticon or Podofilox). Apply to the wart only, avoiding normal skin. Mild burning or irritation is common – if troublesome, the surrounding skin may be masked with vaseline before use. Apply 0.5% solution or 0.15% cream twice daily on 3 consecutive days weekly for 4 weeks. Not recommended if pregnant or breast feeding
Imiquimod	Imiquimod 5% cream available as Aldara in packs of 12 sachets. Apply the contents of one sachet to warts and leave overnight, 3 nights per week (Mon, Wed, Fri). Usually causes erythema, less commonly irritation and inflammation. Each cycle is of 4 weeks, response often takes 8 or more weeks

Box 7.5: Treatment of genital warts

Clinical presentation	Therapy (cryo=liquid nitrogen cryotherapy, pod= podophyllotoxin 0.5% solution or 0.15% cream)
Fleshy, non-keratinized external genital warts, less than six in number	First-line: cryo or pod Second-line: change to alternative (cryo–pod/pod–cryo) Third-line: imiquimod or excision
Papular or keratinized external genital warts	First-line: cryo or cryo/pod alternate weeks Second-line: excision or ablative therapy
Fleshy, non-keratinized external genital warts, more than six in number	First-line: pod Second-line: imiquimod Third-line: ablative therapy
Perianal warts	First-line: cryo or pod Second-line: imiquimod Third-line: surgical resection under general anaesthetic
Vaginal warts	No treatment, cryo or CO_2 laser
Intrameatal warts	First-line: cryo or pod Second-line: electrocautery
Intra-anal warts	No treatment or surgical resection under general anaesthetic
Cervical warts	No treatment (treat any external warts and re-examine for spontaneous resolution). Lletz loop if persist after external lesions resolve

Case study

Lauren (18 years) presented with vulval lumps, itch and an increase in discharge. She had been with her current male partner for 5 months. The lumps had been present for several weeks before she attended a clinic. Examination revealed vulval condylomata acuminata. Investigations showed candidal infection: once this was treated the itch resolved. She was then supplied with podophyllotoxin 0.15% cream. After 10 weeks of 3-day per week therapy two small pedunculated warts remained; these were removed by scissor excision under local anaesthetic. Initially she was distressed by the diagnosis and had avoided sex for weeks. She and her boyfriend were seen together by a health adviser at her second attendance and advised that neither abstinence nor initiating condom use were likely to affect the clinical outcome.

CONDOM USE

With any new partner, or a partner with whom sex has previously been protected, use condoms while warts are being treated and for 6 months after clearance. (The choice of 6 months is arbitrary and the evidence isn't robust.)

With a partner with whom sex regularly took place without a condom before warts appeared, there is no benefit in starting to use condoms.

Condom use is recommended with new partners, but there is little evidence that condoms prevent transmission.

PARTNER NOTIFICATION

As HPV infection is highly prevalent and usually asymptomatic, there is no benefit in tracing current or past sexual partners.

MOLLUSCUM CONTAGIOSUM

BACKGROUND

Mollusum contagiosum is a harmless condition caused by a pox virus. The virus is transmitted through social contact in children, in whom lesions appear on the face, arms and trunk. In adults, sexual transmission is thought to be common: lesions appear on the genitals, sometimes occur in sexual partners, and incidence peaks concurrent with other STIs. Mollusca are rarely a serious clinical problem except in patients with HIV infection, where in advanced immunosuppression they may be extensive, intractable and become secondarily infected.

CLINICAL FEATURES

Incubation is a week to 6 months. Molluscum start as tiny papules, developing a central umbilication as they reach a few millimetres in diameter. Usually multiple lesions at different stages of development can be seen, affecting the genitalia, pubic area, lower abdomen, buttocks and thighs (Fig. 7.9). They do not affect the palms or soles. If lesions

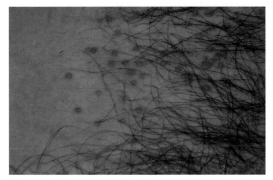

Figure 7.9
Molluscum contagiosum

are seen on the face or neck, consider the possibility of HIV infection. Giant lesions are rare except in the immunosuppressed. Each lesion resolves in a few months: an outbreak usually lasts a few months, occasionally up to 4 years.

DIAGNOSIS

Typical lesions are usually easily recognized. Clinical diagnosis is adequate in immunocompetent patients. A mass of whitish macerated material – a 'core', can be extracted with the tip of a sterile needle and small forceps. Electron microscopy of the core material to demonstrate pox virus, or histological examination of a biopsied lesion may be useful if the diagnosis is in doubt, or in those with immunosuppression. Adults with molluscum contagiosum should always be offered testing for other STIs.

TREATMENT

Destruction of the individual lesions by extraction of the core with a needle or forceps, curettage, cryotherapy or trichloroacetic acid is effective. This can be quite time-consuming and as new lesions may appear over months or years, a single treatment is rarely curative. Podophyllotoxin 0.5% solution or 0.15% cream (as used for wart treatment – see Box 7.5) is useful as patient-applied therapy. There is no truly effective therapy in people with AIDS, but the improvement in cellular immunity with effective antiretroviral therapy may bring spontaneous resolution.

PATIENT INFORMATION

- It is a self-limiting condition.
- It may be sexually transmitted, but good evidence for other modes of transmission. This may be particularly important in regular relationships with children in the household.
- Treatment is for cosmetic reasons only.

ARTHROPOD INFECTIONS

Pediculosis pubis and scabies are arthropod infections, often rather emotively termed 'infestations' for no good reason, affecting the genital skin and hair. Patients with body lice and head lice may also occasionally present to sexual health clinics.

PEDICULOSIS PUBIS

Pthiriasis (pediculosis pubis, crab lice) is caused by the blood-sucking louse *Phthirus pubis* and is usually transmitted by close body contact. Although lice can survive for 24 hours or more away from the human skin, they do not usually leave the host, so transmission through sharing beds or clothing is possible but unlikely.

Clinical features

Sensitivity to the lice is very variable; some patients present with severe itch when only one or two lice can be seen. In others a substantial population of lice is noted in someone with little or no itch. Lice and eggs (nits) may be seen on the pubic hairs, perianal, abdomen or leg hair. Occasionally the eyebrows and eyelashes are affected.

Diagnosis

The lice can be identified by the naked eye, or if necessary with a hand lens. Blue spots (maculae coeuleae) may be seen where the louse has bitten the skin (Fig. 7.10). Patients should be offered tests for other STIs.

Treatment

Head lice (*Pediculus humanus*) develop resistance to the insecticides used for treatment in children. Available treatments are used in rotation in the population in an attempt to avoid the problem. There is no evidence that *Pthirus pubis* has developed resistance to the same pediculocides, but the availability of treatment in any particular area will vary over

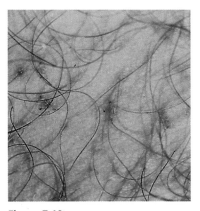

Figure 7.10
Pthiriasis of pubic hair

Box 7.6: Treatment of pediculosis pubis

Permethrin 1%	Apply to damp hair and wash off after 10 minutes
Malathion 0.5%	Leave on for at least 2 hours, preferably overnight. Aqueous emulsion is preferable to alcoholic solution, which is an irritant
Carbaryl 0.5% or 1%	Leave on for at least 2 hours, preferably overnight. Aqueous emulsion is preferable to alcoholic solution, which is an irritant

time. Treatment (Box 7.6) is applied to the skin from the jaw line down, concentrating especially on the hairy areas of the body and including the beard or moustache if present. Eyelashes can be treated by manual removal of lice with forceps or application of vaseline. Clothes and bedding should be washed normally. Repeat treatment after a week, to ensure any newly hatched lice are dealt with.

Patient information

- Usually, but not exclusively sexually transmitted.
- Partners should be treated regardless of symptoms.

SCABIES

Scabies is caused by the mite *Sarcoptes scabiei*. Scabies is transmitted by skin-to-skin contact and at least 20 minutes of contact are thought to be required for transfer of the parasite. Although sexual transmission occurs, outbreaks in families and local epidemics, where transmission is by social contact, have been reported. Symptoms are due to hypersensitivity to the faeces deposited by the mite as it burrows through the stratum corneum.

Clinical features

The main symptom is of severe, distracting itch, worse at night, occurring 2–6 weeks after acquiring infection. Onset is faster in re-infection. Burrows caused by the mites affect the finger webs, wrists, elbows and genitals. Excoriated papules, raised linear burrows and occasionally nodules are seen. The hypersensitivity reaction to the mite faeces may be removed from the site of infection, causing an erythematous urticarial rash affecting the flanks, axillae and upper thighs. Occasionally, secondary bacterial infection occurs complicating the clinical picture. In those with immunosuppression or reduced skin sensation, very large numbers of mites are carried in crusted or Norwegian scabies.

Diagnosis

Clinical diagnosis depends on the recognition of the typical linear burrow ending in a small vesicle. A hand lens and needle can be used to remove the mite from a burrow, or the surface of the whole length of a burrow can be removed with a scalpel. This may be time consuming as some individuals carry very few mites.

Box 7.7: Treatment of scabies

Permethrin 5% cream	Apply to the whole body surface including the scalp. Wash off after 8–12 hours. Reapply to hands if washed within 8 hours of application
Malathion 0.5%	Leave on for at least 2 hours, preferably overnight. Aqueous emulsion is preferable to alcoholic solution, which is an irritant

Treatment

Topical treatments (Box 7.7) are applied to the whole body, including all skin folds, finger webs and under the finger nails. Itch may be severe and persist for weeks after therapy: antihistamines or crotamiton give symptomatic relief and dissuade patients from repeatedly retreating themselves, believing the infection to persist. Clothes and bedding should be washed normally. Sexual and household contacts should also be treated. Oral ivermectin is effective in scabies, but is usually reserved for treatment failure or Norwegian scabies.

OTHER INFECTIVE CONDITIONS

BACTERIAL INFECTIONS

Streptococcal or staphylococcal folliculitis is common and may be precipitated by shaving. It may occasionally be confused with herpes virus infection, but the perifollicular lesions can usually be distinguished. Treatment is with oral flucloxacillin or topical fucidic acid ointment. Similar rashes are seen with furunculosis, hydradenitis and secondarily infected scabies. Bacterial infection with Gram-negative organisms or Vincent's bacteria may cause a balanitis with discharge and offensive smell, particularly in men with phimosis.

FUNGAL INFECTIONS

Candida causes a vulvitis in women (Ch. 3) and balanitis in men. An external or subpreputial swab for microscopic examination and/or culture on Sabouraud's medium should be used to confirm the diagnosis. Dermatophyte infection of the groin (tinea cruris) may occur in isolation or with tinca pcdis. An itchy rash spreads from the groin fold (Fig. 7.11), usually with scaling at the margin, which becomes more erythematous after bathing. A skin scraping or the edge of a dry lesion can be suspended in 10% potassium hydroxide for microscopy, or a scraping or sellotape swab may be cultured. Treatment with an imidazole cream (see Ch. 3) is effective, but eradication can be difficult. Recommend that cream is used twice daily until the lesions resolve and for at least 2 weeks afterwards.

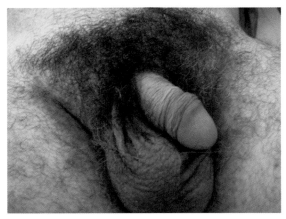

Figure 7.11
Fungal infection of the groin

BALANOPOSTHITIS

Balanoposthitis refers to inflammation of the glans and foreskin secondary to a variety of conditions. Men may present with symptoms of pain or itch, or having noticed a change in appearance with no other symptoms. It is very common for patients to be concerned that the condition is due to sexually transmitted infection. STIs are rarely the cause of balanitis (Fig. 7.12), although *Trichomonas vaginalis*, herpes simplex and syphilis are possible causes. Men sometimes develop balanitis following sex with a new or symptomatic regular partner, suggesting that the acquisition of yeasts, anaerobic bacteria or *Gardnerella vaginalis* during intercourse (see Ch. 3) may be the cause in some cases. However, these organisms are also found in asymptomatic men. Investigation includes:

- testing for sexually transmitted infections (see Ch. 1)
- a subpreputial swab for bacterial culture (Amies)
- a swab or double-sided sticky tape sample for Gram-stain microscopy for the immediate diagnosis of yeast infection
- urinalysis for glucose
- specific tests for ulceration if present (Ch. 6)
- biopsy if the diagnosis is unclear.

Saline bathing is recommended in mild cases: bathing the penis with the foreskin retracted, in 0.9% saline, two or three times per day. In other cases, it is reasonable to give empirical treatment rather than waiting for test results. Erythema, peeling of the skin and longitudinal fissuring of the foreskin suggests yeast infection and can be treated with an imidazole cream, or combined imidazole and steroid. Marked erythema, swelling and a noticeable smell, with mixed organisms on a Gram-stained subpreputial sample is likely to be anaerobic infection and respond to metronidazole.

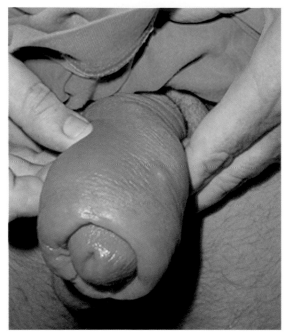

Figure 7.12
Balanitis with oedema of the prepuce

Checklist: differential diagnosis of balanitis

STI: *Trichomonas vaginalis*, HSV, syphilis

Bacterial non-STI: Streptococci, staphylococci, Vincent's organism, anaerobes

Fungal non-STI: *Candida* spp.

Non-infective: Fixed drug eruption, Stevens–Johnson syndrome, allergy, plasma cell balanitis,
                        erythroplasia of Queyrat, lichen sclerosus, trauma, chemical irritant

NON-INFECTIVE CONDITIONS

Dermatitis, lichen planus and psoriasis may affect the genital skin in isolation, or as part of disease affecting the whole of the skin surface. The correct diagnosis of skin disease doesn't exclude STI and some STIs (particularly syphilis) can imitate non-infective skin conditions, so an STI screen is usually appropriate.

CONTACT ALLERGIC DERMATITIS

Cosmetics, soaps, antiseptics, rubber, fabric softeners, topical antibiotics and antifungals may cause contact dermatitis. An acute reaction is often seen within a few hours of contact. The condition may be localized, for example to the glans, causing a balanitis, or affect the whole of the genitalia. Treatment is identification and avoidance of the trigger and moderately potent steroid cream.

LICHEN PLANUS

The lesions of lichen planus (Fig. 7.13) are flat-topped violaceous polygonal papules and are usually itchy. Lesions on the plantar aspect of the wrists or in the mouth support the diagnosis. The disease is self-limiting but a potent steroid cream can be used.

PSORIASIS

Psoriasis may appear as scaling plaques (Fig. 7.14) with an erythematous base on the shaft of the penis or vulva. Psoriatic lesions on the elbows or nail pitting or onycholysis will confirm the diagnosis but genital lesions may occur in isolation. On the glans penis, shiny red lesions without scaling occur and both the macroscopic appearance and histology are indistinguishable from that of circinate balanitis (Ch. 5). Treatment with a mild-to-moderate steroid cream is usually effective.

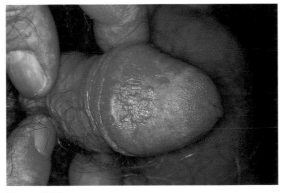

Figure 7.13
Lichen planus

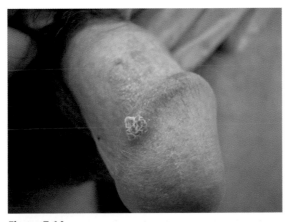

Figure 7.14
Psoriasis

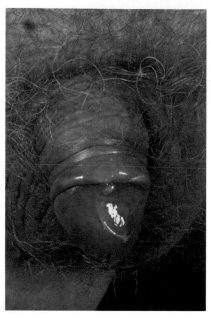

Figure 7.15
Plasma cell balanitis

PLASMA CELL BALANITIS (OF ZOON)

An often painless condition of uncircumcised men, usually over 40 years of age (Fig. 7.15). The aetiology is unknown, but a dysfunction of the foreskin has been suggested. A shiny, red, slightly depressed lesion with a clear margin develops on the glans and/or prepuce. Treatment with Trimovate cream (clobetasone butyrate, nystatin, oxytetracycline) or circumcision is curative in some cases.

FIXED DRUG ERUPTION

Local cutaneous reactions to a variety of drugs may manifest as dusky erythematous patches on the genitals (usually the glans penis). In severe cases, bullae form and the condition is indistinguishable from bullous erythema multiforme.

LICHEN SCLEROSUS

Lichen sclerosus (LS) is a common disease, probably with an autoimmune origin, affecting the genital skin of men and women (Figs 7.16, 7.17, 7.18). In women, atrophic, classically porcelein-white lesions affect the labia minora, clitoral hood, perineum and perianal area. Ecchymoses and telangectasia are common and abrasions and fissures secondary to loss of skin elasticity may also feature. Itch may be severe and atrophy and narrowing of the introitus may cause dyspareunia. Peaks of incidence occur in prepubertal girls and postmenopausal women. In men, the lesions usually affect the glans penis and prepuce (balanitis xerotica obliterans). Scarring of the foreskin causes phimosis and of the glans may cause urethral stenosis. Clinical diagnosis is usually adequate. There is a small

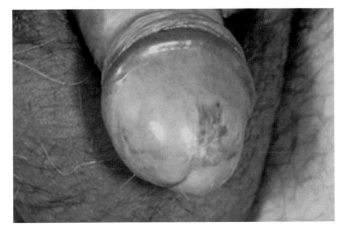

Figure 7.16
Lichen sclerosus of the glans penis

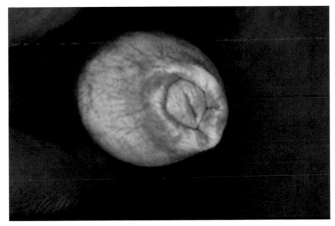

Figure 7.17
Lichen sclerosus affecting the foreskin (balanitis xerotica obliterans)

but definite increase in the risk of squamous carcinoma in women, and probably also in men with LS. Treatment is with the ultrapotent steroid clobetasol propionate (Dermovate), applied once a night for 4 weeks then reducing in frequency over 2 further months. Surgery including circumcision in both sexes may be considered but does not stop the disease process.

LICHEN SIMPLEX (Fig. 7.19)

Scratching or rubbing of the skin, often the vulva or the scrotum, results in erythema and scaling and occasionally to dramatic plaques of lichenification. A course of moderately potent steroid cream may break the 'itch–scratch' cycle and help the condition to settle.

NON-INFECTIVE ULCERS

Sexually transmitted causes of ulceration are discussed in Chapter 6 and should always be considered in the differential diagnosis.

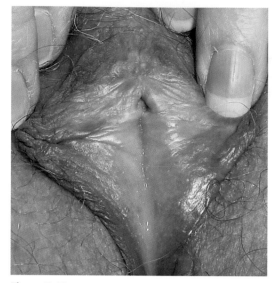

Figure 7.18
Lichen sclerosus of the vulva with atrophy and scarring

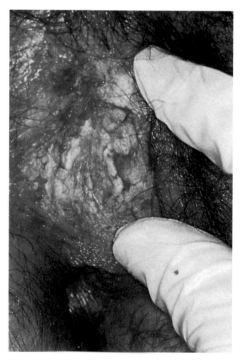

Figure 7.19
Lichen simplex

Bullous erythema multiforme

The severe bullous form of erythema multiforme (also called erythema muliforme exuditavum or Stevens–Johnson syndrome) may affect the genitals as well as the mouth (Fig. 7.20). Important causes include herpes simplex virus, mycoplasmas and drugs, including newer antidepressants. The lesions have an erythematous base covered with white or yellow slough and are surprisingly painless. The classic macular target lesions affecting the extremities may support the diagnosis. Treatment is with strong topical steroids, although systemic steroids should be used if ocular, renal or respiratory involvement occurs.

Behçet's syndrome

This disease is characterized by recurrent episodes of painful oral ulceration in combination with genital ulcers (Fig. 7.21), skin lesions (ulcers, nodules, pustules, erythema nodosum), ocular features (anterior or posterior uveitis, vitreous cellular infiltration) and sometimes arthritis or neurological complications. The underlying lesion is a vasculitis. The diagnosis is made on clinical grounds and is more common in males and in people of Mediterranean and Middle Eastern origin. Proposed diagnostic criteria include the presence of:

- at least three episodes of oral ulceration in a twelve-month period

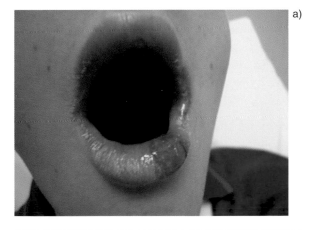
a)

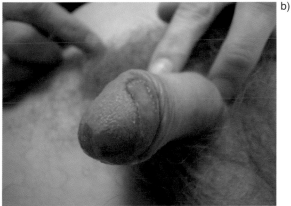
b)

Figure 7.20a,b
Bullous erythema multiforme (oral and penile lesions)

175

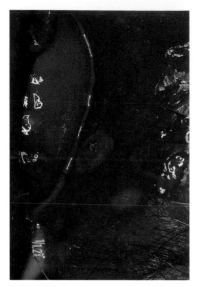

Figure 7.21
Vulval ulceration in Behçet's syndrome

Plus two of the following:

- Recurrent genital apthous ulcers or evidence of scarring
- Eye lesions (uveitis, cells in the vitreous or retinal vasculitis)
- Skin lesions (erythema nodosum, pseudofolliculitis, acneiform lesions)
- Positive pathergy test (hyperreactivity to a needleprick).

Oral and genital apthous ulceration without other manifestations is not uncommon. Strong topical steroids may resolve genital and oral ulcers, but systemic treatment is required in cases with multisystem complications.

Other ulcers

Other non-infective causes of genital ulcers include pyoderma gangrenosum and inflammatory bowel disease, in which genital ulcers may predate gastrointestinal symptoms. Lichen sclerosus may occasionally cause ulceration and premalignant and malignant lesions may ulcerate. Biopsy of any ulcer of unknown aetiology is indicated.

PREMALIGNANT AND MALIGNANT CONDITIONS OF THE GENITALIA

Squamous intraepithelial lesions (Fig. 7.22) of the genitalia may present as macules, plaques, warty lesions or ulcers. Any atypical lesion or undiagnosed ulcer should be biopsied, as should those that fail to resolve with initial therapy.

ERYTHROPLASIA OF QUEYRAT

Well-defined velvety plaques on the glans penis or prepuce, sometimes indistinguishable from plasma cell balanitis of Zoon, characterize this condition. Histologically, it is a

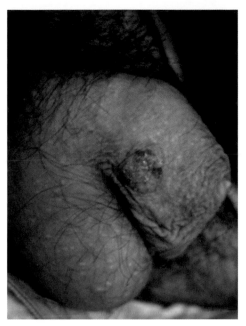

Figure 7.22
Squamous intraepithelial lesion of the penis

squamous-cell carcinoma in situ. Treatment with ablative or antimitotic agents, or excision, is effective.

SQUAMOUS CELL CARCINOMA

Squamous cell carcinomas of the penis and vulva are rare cancers (Fig. 7.23). However, it is not unusual for patients to conclude that such a lesion is related to an STI so they are occasionally seen in GUM clinics.

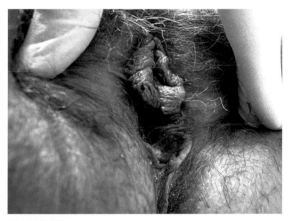

Figure 7.23
Vulval squamous carcinoma

Further Reading

Beuter KR, Wiley DJ, Douglas JM et al. Genital warts and their treatment. Clin Infect Dis 1999; 28 : S37–56.

Birley HDL. Continuing medical ignorance: Modern myths in the management of genital warts. Int Jour STD & AIDS 2001; 12: 71–74.

Brentjens MH, Yeng-Yue KA, Lee PC, Tyring SK. Human papillomavirus: a review. Dermatologic Clinics 2002; 20: 315–331.

Champion RH, Burton JL, Burns DA, Breathnach SM (eds). Textbook of dermatology. Oxford; Blackwell Science: 1998.

Edwards S. Balanitis and balanoposthitis: a review. Genitourin Med 1995; 72: 155–159.

International Study Group for Behçet's disease. Criteria for the diagnosis of Behçet's disease. Lancet 1990; 335:1078–1080.

McMillan A. The management of difficult anogenital warts. Sex Transm Infect 1999; 75:192–194.

Neill SM, Tatnall FM, Cox NH. Guidelines for the management of lichen sclerosus. Br J Dermatol 2002; 147: 640–649.

PHLS, DHSS & PS and the Scottish ISD(D)5 Collaborative Group. Sexually transmitted infections in the UK: New episodes seen at genitourinary medicine clinics, 1991–2001. London; Public Health Laboratory Service: 2002.

SELF-ASSESSMENT

Steven (24 years) is referred by his GP with perianal warts. They have been present for at least 6 months. He is terse and unhappy and says he 'just wants them sorted'. He does not want tests for other infections.

He avoided consulting with his doctor because he was embarrassed. He now has severe perianal itch and some bleeding on defaecation. On examination he has extensive perianal warts, with surrounding erythema, scaling and excoriation.

Questions
a) What avenues could a doctor, nurse or health adviser explore to explain the apparent impact of the problem and deal with his concerns?
b) Suggest a management plan.

Answers
a) His attitude may of course have nothing to do with the warts. However, some of the commoner misconceptions and adverse effects of a diagnosis of warts would be worth exploring the following:
  • What does he know about warts – if anything? Establish understanding of asymptomatic carriage, transmission. Effect on future partners or a current partner. Is he concerned about a past, current or potential future partner? Explain the likelihood that any partner who passed the wart virus on to him was unaware of the infection.
  • Effects on his life, particularly relationships. People sometimes end relationships as a result of an STI diagnosis, wrongly assuming infidelity.
  • Worries about site of warts. He can be reassured that perianal warts often occur in heterosexual men.
  • Why doesn't he want tests for infection? Is it fear of examination and swab taking, or concern about the possible results? Explain the possibility of having other asymptomatic infections.
b) The warts are likely to be secondarily infected. An attempt can be made to diagnose fungal infection from skin scrapings from the edge of the erythematous area. Alternatively empirical treatment with clotrimazole cream, or if the warts are 'boggy' and macerated, topical eosin 2% solution, may be used prior to treatment for warts. Treatment with podophyllotoxin cream, imiquimod cream or cryotherapy would be appropriate. For extensive perianal warts, some clinicians would use imiquimod 5% cream as first line therapy.

Viral hepatitis and the management of blood-borne virus exposure

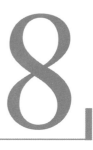

BACKGROUND

Although viral hepatitis may be sexually transmitted, presentation with acute hepatitis is relatively uncommon in sexual health clinics. More commonly, patients are offered vaccination because of increased risk of infection with hepatitis A or B. Chronic infection with hepatitis B is endemic in much of the world, but in northern Europe and the USA is mainly confined to people originating from endemic areas and those in, or who have contact with, high-risk subgroups such as men who have sex with men (MSM), sex workers and intravenous drug users (IDUs). People in these groups may be tested for antibodies to hepatitis B prior to being offered vaccination if at continued risk. Such testing will identify the minority of at-risk individuals who are already carriers of hepatitis B. These patients require advice on further management and the prevention of onward transmission. Because the modes of transmission of HIV and hepatitis coincide, many patients with HIV infection will also be infected with hepatitis B and/or C. Co-infection further complicates the management of chronic hepatitis and is discussed in Chapter 10. Consensus statements on which asymptomatic at-risk individuals should be tested for hepatitis C infection exist in the USA, UK and France, although the implications of screening are still a subject of debate. Fears regarding employment, insurance and other social issues resulting from a diagnosis of hepatitis C are in some ways similar to those that apply to HIV infection (Ch. 9) and for this reason many people in the UK choose to be tested for hepatitis C anonymously. Responsibility for occupational exposure to blood-borne viruses may also fall within the remit of sexual health or GUM services, as may the assessment and follow up of those exposed, or potentially exposed, through sexual assault or rape. Knowledge of the natural history of hepatitis and the issues surrounding testing is, therefore, vital for anyone working in sexual health.

HEPATITIS VIRUSES

Hepatitis viruses may be encountered in sexual healthcare in the following ways (see Box 8.1).

Acute symptomatic illness

Over 80% of cases of acute hepatitis are due to hepatitis A or B, but acute hepatitis may also be caused by the hepatitis viruses C, D and E, by cytomegalovirus (CMV) or Epstein-Barr virus (EBV), and by non-infectious agents.

Box 8.1: Hepatitis viruses in sexual health

	Transmission	Acute hepatitis	Routine testing	Chronic infection	Vaccination available
Hepatitis A	Faeco-oral Sexual (MSM: oro-anal or digital–anal contact) (Blood-to-blood rare)	yes	yes	no	yes
Hepatitis B	Vertical Blood-to-blood Sexual (mucous membrane shedding)	yes	yes	yes	yes
Hepatitis C	Blood-to-blood (Sexual rare) (Vertical rare)	yes	yes	yes	no
Hepatitis D	Blood-to-blood Sexual (thought rare)	yes	no	yes	no (though hepatitis B vaccination is protective)
Hepatitis E	Faeco-oral	yes	no	no	no

Symptomatic or asymptomatic chronic infection

Chronic infection with hepatitis B (HBV) or hepatitis C (HCV) may lead to complications including cirrhosis and hepatocellular carcinoma. The management of chronic infection is not covered here, although information relevant to the testing and counselling of patients with chronic infection is included.

Vaccination of those at risk of infection

Vaccination against hepatitis A and B is commonly offered in parts of the world where the infections aren't endemic. In some nations, universal vaccination for hepatitis B is practiced. In others (including UK) vaccination is offered only to those regarded as being at increased risk of infection.

PATHOGENESIS AND CLINICAL PRACTICE

Hepatitides A to E are caused by unrelated viruses with few similarities in epidemiology or pathogenesis. Virtually their only common 'family' characteristics are overlapping modes of transmission and affinity for the hepatocyte.

Hepatitis A and E do not possess a lipid envelope and are excreted intact from infected liver cells into the bile where they can survive and pass into the gastrointestinal tract. Consequently, they are spread by faeco–oral contamination. Sexual transmission is involved in a minority of infections, usually in MSM. These viruses do not cause persistent infection.

Hepatitis B, C and D are covered by a lipid-containing envelope and are inactivated by bile, so are not excreted in the gut. Transmission of these viruses is by blood-to-blood or mucous membrane exposure.

Hepatitis A

Common in countries with poor sanitation, where immunity to hepatitis A approaches 100% in young adults. With reducing prevalence in developed nations, a common cause of illness in travellers. In low prevalence populations, hepatitis A occurs in MSM, associated with oro–anal or digital–anal sexual contact and with multiple and anonymous partners. Large-scale urban outbreaks also occur affecting all age groups and sectors of the population, with household contact and contact with children in day care as significant risk factors. Seroprevalence in homosexual and heterosexual men in non-endemic populations is the same and it is not clear whether vaccination should be recommended on the grounds of sexual orientation. Hepatitis A outbreaks occur in intravenous drug users (IVDUs), although whether this relates to poor sanitation, or whether the virus is transmitted through blood–blood contact during acute infection has not been ascertained.

Symptom severity increases with age, and children under 5 years are almost always asymptomatic. Full recovery occurs in 3 months in 85% of adult cases. Fulminant hepatitis develops in 0.4% and is fatal in 0.2%, although risk is higher in the elderly. Chronic carriage does not occur.

Hepatitis B

Hepatitis B is highly transmissible by mucous membrane contact during peno–anal and peno–vaginal sex and parturition. It is endemic in much of the world where carrier rates are up to 20%. Transmission in Africa is mostly vertical; in SE Asia, where the mode of transmission is incompletely understood, it is horizontal in the first year of life. Rates of transmission to the sexual partners of carriers, and vertical transmission rates are high. Vertical transmission rate is 90% if a mother is HbsAg and HbeAg positive. Acute symptomatic illness is rare in children, but over 90% develop chronic infection. Adults in non-endemic settings such as UK and USA, where seroprevalence is 0.01–1%, are at risk if MSM, sex workers, IVDUs or contacts of carriers. In southern and eastern Europe, prevalence rates are 2–5%. HBV survives for at least a week in dried blood spills, which may explain outbreaks in health-care workers without history of needlestick injury. In acute infection symptomatic illness occurs in up to 50% of adults but less than 5% become chronic carriers. Fulminant hepatitis develops in fewer than 1% of cases, but is commoner with hepatitis C co-infection.

Hepatitis C

Worldwide, the prevalence of hepatitis C infection is five times that of HIV, affecting at least 170 million people. In developed nations, even though only a tiny minority of those infected are aware of their infection, chronic hepatitis C is the most common indication for liver transplantation. Acute symptomatic illness is rare, but fatality from fulminant hepatic failure is reported in up to 2.5% of symptomatic cases. Chronic carriage occurs in

8.5% of those infected. Prevalence varies widely throughout the world, and in different risk populations. No vaccine is available.

In the UK, seroprevalence is less than 1% in blood donors but up to 85% in intravenous drug users (Fig. 8.1). Transmission in non-endemic settings occurs through blood–blood contact (shared needles in inravenous drug users, contaminated blood products prior to 1991), which is very highly efficient. The annual incidence of infection in people newly injecting intravenous drugs is 5–28%. Mucous membrane transmission is much less efficient so the rate of sexual transmission is low (0.2–2% per year of regular relationship) and vertical transmission is uncommon (5%). However, co-infection with HIV and hepatitis C appears to substantially increase the transmission of hepatitis C by these routes.

Hepatitis D

An incomplete virus incapable of transmission in the absence of hepatitis B. It may co-infect an individual simultaneously with acute hepatitis B infection, or cause an acute hepatitis when superinfection occurs in a chronic hepatitis B carrier. Fulminant hepatitis and death may occur in either situation, and chronic infection is more likely than with HBV alone, carrying an increased risk of complications. Co-infection rate with HDV in HBsAg +ve carriers of HBV is higher in IVDU than in MSM or heterosexual individuals. This is consistent with the theory that sexual transmission is possible but uncommon. HBV vaccination protects against both HBV and HDV. No vaccine to protect against superinfection with HDV is available for chronic carriers of hepatitis B infection.

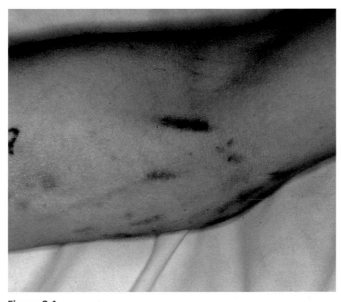

Figure 8.1
Needle tracks in an intravenous drug user

Hepatitis E

Similar to Hepatitis A, transmission is by the oro–faecal route. Outbreaks of 100s to tens of thousands of cases have been reported. Mortality may be up to 20% in pregnant women. Sexual transmission is not reported. Chronic infection does not occur.

Hepatitis G

Hepatitis G virus (HGV) is also known as GB virus C. It rarely causes acute hepatitis. Persistent infection occurs but without hepatitis. HGV co-infection may have a protective effect against progression of HIV infection.

ACUTE HEPATITIS

CLINICAL FEATURES

An incubation period (variable according to the infecting virus – see Box 8.2) is followed in the classic case by prodromal symptoms and then an icteric illness. However, up to half of adults and virtually all children under 5 years have a mild non-specific illness or are asymptomatic.

In symptomatic patients the prodrome consists of flu-like symptoms lasting for around a week. 30–70% of adults and older children with acute viral hepatitis then develop jaundice, anorexia and nausea lasting 1–3 weeks. Jaundice is more common in those acquiring hepatitis B or C through i.v. drug use than through other modes of transmission (Fig. 8.2) and is more severe in hepatitis B than hepatitis A. Severe illness is also likely when acute hepatitis occurs as superinfection (such as HDV superinfection of a chronic HBV carrier or acute HBV infection in a chronic HCV carrier). Symptoms and signs are not helpful in distinguishing the causative virus type in acute hepatitis, so clinical suspicion in the symptomatic patient should trigger full examination and diagnostic tests.

Box 8.2: Clinical features of acute hepatitis

	Incubation period Mean (range) in days	Complications of acute illness	Infectious period	Other features
Hepatitis A	30 (15–50)	Prolonged cholestasis (jaundice lasting several weeks) Fulminant hepatitis (0.4%)	1 week prior to and two weeks after symptoms	
Hepatitis B	80 (30–160)	Serum sickness Pancreatitis Fulminant hepatitis (0.8–4%)	2 weeks prior to jaundice until surface antigen negative	Serum sickness-like illness in 10%; rash and arthralgia
Hepatitis C	50 (15–80)	Fulminant hepatitis		Serum sickness-like illness in 10%; rash and arthralgia

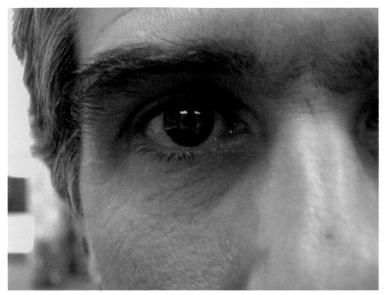

Figure 8.2
Jaundiced sclera in acute Hepatitis B

History

The clinical history should include a standard sexual history plus details of place of birth and ethnic origin, recent travel, employment, injections, blood transfusion and symptoms in household and sexual contacts. Details of alcohol intake, and prescribed and recreational drug use are important in excluding non-infectious causes of hepatitis.

Clinical notes: symptoms of acute hepatitis

- Nausea and vomiting
- Change in smell or taste
- Fatigue or malaise
- Right upper-quadrant pain
- Diarrhoea
- Itch (may indicate cholestasis).

Examination

Do a full systemic examination, including assessment of consciousness level and for signs of encephalopathy in ill or jaundiced patients. Undertake routine screening for STIs as described in Chapter 1: if the patient is admitted to hospital, this may otherwise be overlooked as the acute illness is managed.

Signs

- None in prodromal phase
- Jaundice
- Hepatomegaly (may be tender) (10%)

185

- Splenomegaly (5%)
- Lymphadenopathy (5%)
- No signs of chronic liver disease (if there are signs of chronic liver disease, consider superinfection – see above).

INVESTIGATIONS

Alanine transaminase (ALT) and asparate aminotransferase (AST), markers of liver injury, are increased at least 8× upper limit of normal (ULN) and may be increased several hundred-fold. Dramatic increases in ALT and AST in the acute phase do not necessarily indicate poor prognosis.

Alkaline phosphatase and bilirubin are increased only 2–3-fold unless the illness is complicated by cholestasis. Amylase, creatinine kinase (CK) and lactate dehydrogenase (LDH) are usually normal or increased less than 3-fold. Note that hepatitis B occasionally presents with pancreatitis.

Full blood count parameters are usually only mildly deranged. There may be a lymphocytosis, mild anaemia or thrombocytopenia.

Prothrombin time (PT) – any increase in PT greater than 5 seconds or INR greater than 2 signifies incipient liver failure and indicates the need for admission and close monitoring.

Serological tests in acute hepatitis

Initial serological tests may depend on local availability (see Box 8.3). Baseline tests may include:

Box 8.3: Serological tests in acute hepatitis

Test		Comments
HAV IgM	IgM antibody to hepatitis A virus	Diagnostic of acute hepatitis A
HBsAg	Hepatitis B surface antigen	Acute hepatitis B or hepatitis B chronic carrier Detectable 2–12 weeks after infection. May occasionally be cleared from serum by the time the patient presents with jaundice
IgM Anti-HBc	IgM antibody to hepatitis B core antigen	Diagnostic of acute hepatitis B
IgG Anti-HBc	IgG antibody to hepatitis B core antigen	Positive in acute and chronic hepatitis B
HBeAg	Hepatitis B e antigen.	Detectable in acute hepatitis B and chronic carriage of high infectivity
Anti-HBe	Hepatitis B e antibody (anti-HBe)	Resolving acute hepatitis B infection or chronic carrier, low infectivity
HBV DNA	Hepatitis B viral DNA	Detectable in acute hepatitis B and chronic carriage of high infectivity
Anti-HDV	Antibody to hepatitis D	Acute or chronic hepatitis D infection Detectable 1–2 months after infection
HDV RNA	Hepatitis D viral RNA	Acute hepatitis D infection

- Hepatitis A IgM antibody (HAV IgM)
- Hepatitis B surface antigen (HBsAg)
- Hepatitis B e antigen (HBeAg)
- Hepatitis B IgG core antibody (IgG Anti-HBc)
- Hepatitis B IgM core antibody (IgM Anti-HBc).

Some laboratories may offer a single screening test for hepatitis B, usually hepatitis B surface antigen (HBsAg) and undertake further tests only if this is positive.

Case history

Laurence (23 years) attended the GUM clinic for the first time on the advice of a friend. He had had unprotected insertive and receptive oral sex with around 50 men in the previous 3 months. He had felt generally unwell with fevers, nausea and myalgia for about a week. There were no abnormal findings on examination. He was tested for sexually transmitted infections including HIV and hepatitis B, and given his first combined hepatitis A and B vaccination. He returned to the clinic the following week with jaundice. The hepatitis B surface antigen result reported from his first visit was positive. His liver function was monitored weekly for the first month. He made a full recovery and HBsAg was negative 3 months later.

Other tests

If first-line tests for hepatitis are negative, or clinical suspicion is high, consider:

- Hepatitis C vRNA
- IgM antibody to Ebstein-Barr virus (EBV IgM)
- IgM antibody to cytomegalovirus (CMV IgM)
- Antibody to hepatitis D (anti-HDV) (hepatitis D superinfection: anti-HDV with hepatitis B surface antigen (HbsAg), but IgM anti-HBc negative)
- Antibody to hepatitis E (IgG Anti-HEV)
- Antinuclear antibody (ANA), anti-smooth muscle antibody, anti-neutrophil antibody (autoimmune hepatitis)
- Serum copper and caeruloplasmin (Wilson's disease)
- Serum ferritin (haemachromatosis).

MANAGEMENT

Antiviral drugs are not currently routinely indicated in the treatment of acute hepatitis. Recently, antivirals such as lamivudine have been used in acute hepatitis B infection. Drug treatment of acute hepatitis C with high-dose interferon has shown some success in clinical trials and may be available in some centres. Previously healthy adults with mild-to-moderate cases of hepatitis can be monitored as outpatients, checking liver function weekly until normal. If illness is severe, cholestasis supervenes or prothrombin time is increased by more than 5 seconds, admit. The development of signs of hepatic encephalopathy within 8 weeks of symptoms first appearing is diagnostic of fulminant hepatic failure and is an indication for immediate referral to a specialist unit. Those with hepatitis A should be followed up until the liver function returns to normal. People with acute hepatitis B should have HBsAg repeated at 6 months to confirm seroreversion, excluding chronic infection.

COUNSELLING, INFORMATION AND PARTNER NOTIFICATION

Acute hepatitis A, B and C are notifiable diseases (UK) and should be notified to the local consultant in communicable disease who can arrange vaccination of household/work contacts. Tracing of sexual contacts is often more appropriately dealt with by sexual health staff.

Partner notification and vaccination

Hepatitis A

Sexual contacts of MSM with hepatitis A in the infectious period (see Box 8.2), household contacts, other contacts if index patient is a food handler: give human normal immunoglobulin 250–500 mg i.m. if within 10 days of their first contact with the patient. Otherwise initiate the standard hepatitis A vaccination schedule (see below).

Hepatitis B

All sexual contacts of both homosexual and heterosexual patients, needle sharing partners in the infectious period (see Box 8.2). See guidance below on hepatitis B vaccination.

Hepatitis C

There is no established intervention for contacts in the acute phase, but needle sharing and recent sexual partners should be offered follow-up for antibody testing 6 months after exposure.

CHRONIC VIRAL HEPATITIS

Patients may be diagnosed with chronic hepatitis infection in the sexual health clinic, so details relevant to initial assessment and counselling patients is included. Treatment is not covered.

CHRONIC HEPATITIS B

Chronic hepatitis B infection may be identified when hepatitis serology is checked prior to, or simultaneous with offering vaccination to people at risk of infection. It is advisable to test for prior exposure to hepatitis in such individuals, most of whom, if they originate from a non-endemic area but have been exposed to hepatitis B as adults, will have cleared infection and be immune. See Box 8.4 for interpretation of hepatitis B serology. The risk of chronic infection is much higher in those born in endemic areas. Those who are exposed but immune to infection will have antibody to hepatitis B core antigen (anti-HBc) but no detectable hepatitis B surface antigen (HBsAg negative) and are not at risk of either transmission to others or to liver damage. A minority of those tested will be chronic carriers of hepatitis B infection with detectable serum hepatitis B surface antigen (HBsAg). Most people with chronic infection do not have a history of jaundice. Chronic

Box 8.4: Interpretation of hepatitis B serology

	HBsAg	Anti-HBs	HBeAg	Anti-HBe	Anti-HBc	Anti-HBcIgM
Acute HBV infection	+	–	+	–	+	+
Previous exposure: immune	–	+/–	–	+/–	+	–
Carrier of low infectivity	+	–	–	+	+	–
Carrier of intermediate infectivity	+	–	–	–	+	–
Carrier of high infectivity	+	–	+	–	+	–
Vaccine induced immunity	–	+	–	–	–	–

Note HBcAg is found in the liver but not in the blood

carriers of low infectivity with little or no liver inflammation will have antibody to hepatitis B 'e' antigen (Anti-HBe), no detectable hepatitis B 'e' antigen (HBeAg negative), normal ALT and low levels of hepatitis B DNA. Others will have high levels of HBV DNA, usually accompanied by positive hepatitis B 'e' antigen (HBeAg) in addition to HBsAg and abnormal liver function. If liver biopsy is done on these people there is evidence of continuing inflammation of the liver, carrying the risk of cirrhosis and its complications. The presence of hepatitis 'e' antigen (HBeAg) is a marker of infectiousness. A precore mutant of hepatitis B exists, which does not appear to produce HBeAg and is associated with a high level of progression to cirrhosis. Infection with precore mutant is associated with HBsAg positivity and high levels of HBV DNA, but negative HBeAg and positive Anti-HBe.

Information of use in counselling and advising patients

Ninety-five per cent of those with HBV infection acquired in adulthood make a complete recovery, whereas 95% of those infected in early childhood will be chronic carriers.

Chronic infection is identified by the presence of HBsAg in the blood 6 months or more after infection. Those with the highest levels of HBV replication, reflected in the HBV DNA level in a quantitative assay, are the most infectious and have the highest risk of long-term complications. These individuals are usually (not always) HBeAg positive.

Up to 80% of those with chronic infection will seroconvert from HBeAg to anti-HBe within 5 years. Delayed seroconversion to anti-HBe is associated with chronic active hepatitis and liver damage. Seroconversion to anti-HBe reduces, but does not abolish the risk of progression.

Ten to 50% of chronic carriers (HBsAg positive) develop cirrhosis, of whom 10% develop hepatocellular carcinoma.

Progression is more rapid in men, in those co-infected with hepatitis C, hepatitis D or HIV, with younger age at acquisition and with alcohol intake.

Carriers with HBsAg who are HBeAg negative and who have undetectable HBV DNA and normal AST are at low risk of complications. Treatment of chronic hepatitis B infection may be considered in those with HBeAg and/or detectable HBV DNA.

Treatment with interferon, lamivudine, famciclovir, adefovir or a combination of drugs can achieve seroreversion and suppress viraemia in up to 50% of patients, reducing the risk of cirrhosis and hepatocellular carcinoma.

Clinical notes: initial management of HBsAg positive hepatitis B carrier

- Check infectivity and risk of complications with full hepatitis B serology: HBsAg, HBeAg, anti-HBe, HBV DNA
- Exclude co-infection with HCV and HDV (co-infection accelerates progression)
- Check liver function, albumin, clotting , alpha FP and USS liver
- Vaccinate against hepatitis A
- Screen and vaccinate sexual partners, children and household contacts
- Advise against blood, semen, organ donation, sharing of injecting equipment
- Advise patient to inform dentists and medical personnel, carers
- If HBeAg positive or detectable HBV DNA refer to specialist unit to consider therapy

CHRONIC HEPATITIS C

Issues relating to the risk of sexual transmission, occupational exposure and informed consent to testing for hepatitis C are covered here.

People with chronic hepatitis C rarely have clinical signs unless advanced cirrhosis or hepatocellular carcinoma is present at presentation. The initial screening test is for hepatitis C antibody. If positive, a PCR for hepatitis C viral RNA will determine whether there is persisting infection. Antibody testing is false negative in 0.5–1% of individuals, but the rate is higher in HIV infection (especially when immunosuppression is advanced), in renal failure and essential mixed cryoglobulinaemia. Treatment of hepatitis C is a rapidly developing field. At present, the best results are achieved with a combination of pegylated interferon as a weekly injection, combined with oral ribavirin. This achieves sustained viral suppression in up to 50% of those with genotype 1 and 80% of those with genotype 2 or 3.

Information of use in counselling and advising patients

A minority of patients infected with hepatitis C clear the virus, developing anti-hepatitis C antibody but no persistent viraemia. Seventy-five per cent to 85% of patients are persistently viraemic with chronic infection. An antibody screening test is routinely used for hepatitis C testing and is usually followed by a PCR test for viral RNA if positive.

Six genotypes of hepatitis C have been identified. Type 1b may be associated with a more rapid progression to cirrhosis. Types 1a and 1b are less likely to respond to therapy.

The majority of those with hepatitis C develop liver inflammation detectable at biopsy. Cirrhosis develops in 15–20% of those infected, of whom 1–4% per year develop hepatocellular carcinoma. About one-third of patients have serious liver disease less than

20 years after infection and one-third are free of cirrhosis for more than 30 years. Around 10% of those chronically infected have symptoms.

Progression is more rapid in men, in those with hepatitis B and HIV co-infection, with age and with alcohol intake. Cessation or reduction of alcohol intake is the only action influencing the course of the disease that is under the patient's control.

Superinfection with hepatitis A can cause a severe, potentially fatal hepatitis in those with HCV. Hepatitis A vaccination is safe and should be initiated soon after diagnosis.

Current recommendations are that liver biopsy is indicated only in those with raised ALT, but this has been questioned as a significant proportion of patients with normal ALT may have cirrhosis.

Clinical notes: initial management of a patient with hepatitis C antibodies

- Hepatitis C antibody EIA screening test positive: confirm with RIBA assay, third-generation ELISA, or hepatitis C vRNA
- Check ALT, AST, bilirubin, INR
- Test for hepatitis viruses: Hepatitis A IgG (anti-HAV), HBcAb, HbsAg
- Discuss HIV testing if not done simultaneously
- Caeruloplasmin, serum copper, ferritin, autoantibody screen
- Vaccinate against hepatitis A and B

HEPATITIS B VACCINATION

Vaccination against hepatitis B with recombinant vaccines appears to be highly effective. Following the introduction of universal vaccination in Taiwan, the prevalence of HbsAg in children fell by over 80% and no hepatocellular carcinomas occurred in children born after the start of the vaccination programme. The World Health Organization recommended universal vaccination should be introduced in all countries by 1997, but this has not been widely adopted. Those at risk of hepatitis B infection in countries where hepatitis B is not endemic include:

- The sexual partners and close household contacts of hepatitis B carriers
- The sexual partners and close household contacts of those with acute hepatitis B
- Babies born to hepatitis B carrier mothers or mothers with acute hepatitis B
- Haemophiliacs and others receiving frequent blood transfusions or blood products
- Homosexual men
- Sex industry workers
- People travelling for extended periods in endemic areas
- Workers in health care, laboratories or institutions
- Prison inmates.

These individuals may be offered hepatitis B vaccination (Fig. 8.3).

Vaccination against hepatitis B will produce an immune response to a recombinant form of HBsAg, measurable as anti-HBs, in 90% of those vaccinated after a course of three

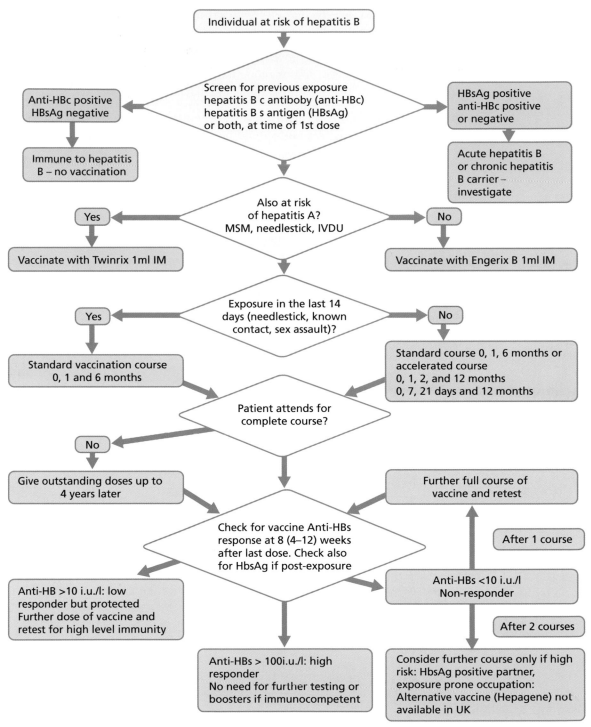

Figure 8.3
Hepatitis B vaccination

injections. Mild side effects are common and include pain at the injection site; more rarely fever or flu-like symptoms. Serious side effects are extremely rare. Pregnancy is not a contraindication to vaccination. The vaccine is given intramuscularly into the deltoid. The vaccines commonly used are Engerix B 1ml IM (hepatitis B only) or Twinrix 1ml IM (combined hepatitis A and B). These may be given at 0, 1 and 6 months followed by a test of response. An accelerated course of 0, 7 and 21 days with a booster at 12 months gives comparable levels of immunity and is increasingly used as the standard dosage regimen because uptake is better. The accelerated course has not been evaluated for post exposure vaccination and the standard course should be used until further evidence is available. People who do not respond to an initial course of vaccination should be given a further full course.

EXPOSURE TO BLOOD-BORNE VIRUSES

Responsibility for the immediate management of occupational and other exposure to blood-borne viruses (BBV) may involve staff in genitourinary medicine, emergency services, occupational health, general practice and other fields. National guidelines exist in the UK and USA for the management of exposure, and in many areas local protocols define lines of responsibility and management guidelines (see Further reading). Familiarize yourself with local procedures and the availability of medication if required. This section deals with the practicalities of dealing with such a situation and should be used in conjunction with published guidelines.

Potential exposure to blood-borne viruses may be through occupational exposure, affecting health-care workers, support workers, those in the emergency services, students, local government workers and volunteers, as well as non-occupational exposure in members of the public occurring as a result of sexual or violent assault or injuries from discarded needles (Fig. 8.4). The term 'blood-borne viruses' in this context includes hepatitis C, hepatitis B and HIV.

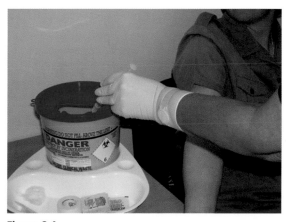

Figure 8.4
Safe disposal of contaminated sharps

ASSESSMENT

Make an immediate and rapid assessment of the exposure, considering the following factors:

1. The extent of exposure: the nature of injury or mucosal or other contact.
2. The body fluid involved: blood, saliva, vomitus, etc.
3. The source (or 'index' or 'donor') case: is the exposure from a source *known to have*, or *thought to be at risk of* infection?

The combination of these factors allows advice to be given on appropriate action. If the exposure is potentially significant, consider hepatitis B, C and HIV in turn (Fig. 8.5). Bear in mind that recent experience suggests that post-exposure prophylaxis has often been given unnecessarily and that most exposures are low risk. The likelihood of seroconversion after needlestick injury is best studied and gives an indication of the risk of other exposures (see Box 8.5). Hepatitis B carries the highest risk of transmission and outbreaks have been attributed to non-penetrating exposure to blood-contaminated surfaces. Hepatitis B may survive on such surfaces (and, theoretically, on a discarded needle), for up to 1 week. It is thought that mucous membrane exposure and non-intact skin exposure carry significant risk of hepatitis B transmission. The risk of HIV transmission through mucous membrane exposure is estimated at 0.09% and transmission through non-intact skin is lower still but has been reported. Transmission of HIV through intact skin has not been documented. Hepatitis C carries the lowest risk of transmission of all, with mucous membrane transmission very rarely reported and no reported transmission through intact or non-intact skin. Risk fluids for BBV infection

Box 8.5: Risk of BBV transmission by nature of contact, with estimates of transmission risk where available

	Needlestick		Mucosal contact (mouth, conjunctiva) Skin contact	Sexual exposure
HIV	0.3% overall Higher risk Hollow needle Blood in bone Deep injury High viral load AIDS	Lower risk Solid needle Passed through glove Effective treatment	Mucous membrane <0.09% Non intact skin <0.01% Intact skin: none reported	Single act: Receptive anal intercourse 0.5–3% Receptive vaginal intercourse 0.01–0.15% Receptive oral sex 0.04% Condom use reduces risk by 80%
Hep C	1.5–3% overall		Mucosal contact: few single case reports, very rare No transmission through intact or non-intact skin	0.2–2% per year in regular relationship Very low from single contact
Hep B	HBsAg and HBeAg positive: 40–60% risk seroconversion 20–30% risk clinical hepatitis HBsAg pos, HBeAg neg: 20–40% risk seroconversion 1–6% risk clinical hepatitis		Mucous membrane and non-intact skin exposure carries risk	40% in sexual partners of people with acute or chronic hepatitis B Single contact risk unknown, likely to be higher than HIV or hep C

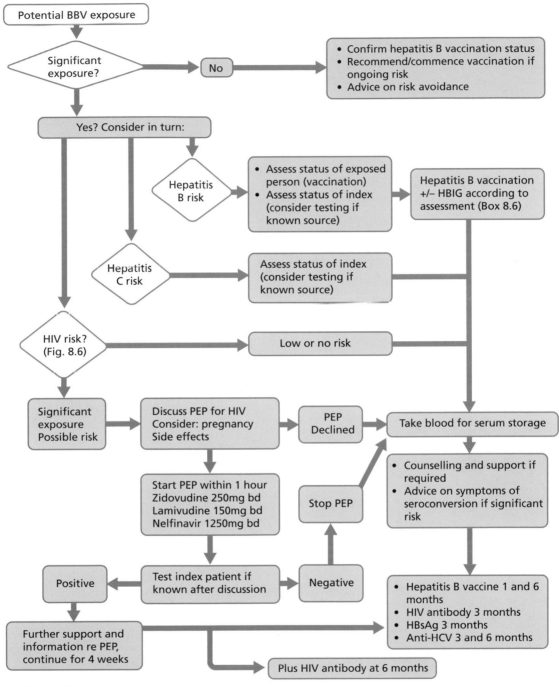

Figure 8.5
Assessment of exposure to hepatitis B, C and HIV

include blood and other body fluids including amniotic, synovial, peritoneal, and pericardial fluids, semen and CSF. Saliva, sputum, sweat, urine and vomitus are not considered infectious.

Hepatitis B exposure

Most healthcare workers have been vaccinated against hepatitis B and will have evidence of immunity. Many other public service workers, such as police and local authority staff in the UK, are not routinely vaccinated.

The risk of transmission from an infected individual is high, but the prevalence of infection in the population of the UK and other non-endemic nations is low. If the source patient is known, consider testing for HBsAg (see below).

Evidence from the treatment of babies born to hepatitis B infected mothers suggests that hepatitis B immunoglobulin (HBIG) plus an immunization course reduces the risk of transmission by about 90%, vaccination alone by 75%.

In most situations a course of hepatitis B vaccination alone is appropriate, unless the index patient is known to be a hepatitis B carrier. There are epidemiological reasons to minimize the routine use of hepatitis B immunoglobulin: it is thought to be a significant factor in the development of vaccine escape mutants in a population. See Box 8.6 for recommendations in specific circumstances.

Box 8.6: Post exposure prophylaxis for hepatitis B exposure

Vaccination/response of person at risk	Source HbsAg positive	Source HbsAg negative	Source status unknown
Never vaccinated or 1 dose only	Vaccination course plus HBIG ×1	Initiate vaccination (non-urgent)	Vaccination course
Known responder to vaccine[1]	No treatment	No treatment	No treatment
Known non-responder to vaccine	HBIG ×1 +/– revaccination[2]	No treatment	If high risk source HBIG ×1 revaccination[2]
Vaccination status or response unknown	Test exposed person for HBsAb and see above[1] or HBIG ×1 and vaccine booster	Arrange routine HBsAb testing and revaccination (non-urgent)	Test exposed person for HBsAb and see above[1]

[1]An individual with HbsAb (serum antibody to hepatitis B surface antigen) level of >10 miU/ml is regarded as a responder and is protected. A level of <10 miU/ml is a non-responder.
[2]If non-responder after one course of vaccine, give HBIG ×1 and restart vaccination course. If non-responder after two courses, give HBIG ×2

(Based on US Public Health Service, 2001)

Hepatitis C exposure

Small trials of post exposure prophylaxis (PEP) for hepatitis C infection with antivirals such as interferon and ribavirin have shown some effect but current USA and UK guidelines do not recommend any form of PEP in this situation. This may change – check the latest guidelines.

HIV exposure

The use of post exposure prophylaxis (PEP) to prevent HIV infection is based on knowledge of HIV pathogenesis, animal studies and limited case-control evidence. Giving antiretroviral drugs soon after an inoculation of virus may prevent viral replication at the initial stage of dendritic cell migration to local lymph nodes and so avert infection (see Ch. 9). Animal studies using simian immunodeficiency virus (SIV), a virus closely related to HIV, in macaques support this theory. A large case-control study of healthcare workers given zidovudine following occupational exposure to HIV suggests that the risk of seroconversion is reduced by 81% compared to those who receive no treatment. Combination therapy is now recommended for post exposure prophylaxis for HIV, based on its superior efficacy in reducing mother-to-child transmission and in the treatment of established HIV infection. In cases where the risk of HIV infection is thought to be significant, a combination of zidovudine, lamivudine and nelfinavir at standard doses (Ch. 11), continued for 4 weeks is recommended in the UK. Indinavir or saquinavir may be used instead of nelfinavir. Other combinations of licensed antiretrovirals may be considered on the grounds of tolerability and in cases where the index patient has previously been exposed and has developed resistance to antiretroviral drugs. Nevirapine is not recommended as a component of PEP because of the very rare possibility of fatal hepatitis. Figure 8.6 may be used in conjunction with published guidelines to make an initial decision on whether PEP for HIV should be given. In cases of exposure to people known to have HIV infection, details of viral load, previous and current antiretroviral therapy and if available, resistance testing results may be useful in deciding on the appropriate regimen. In cases of occupational exposure from a patient of unknown serostatus it is usually appropriate to test the index patient for BBV. A decision on whether to continue PEP can then be made. Some guidance on testing in these circumstances is given below. The aim is to give PEP for HIV within an hour of exposure, so in most cases one or two doses of antiretrovirals will have been given before a result is available. There is some evidence that PEP is effective up to 12 hours after exposure and in cases with very high transmission risk some authorities recommend the use of PEP up to two weeks after exposure.

BBV risk assessment – approaching the index patient

The index or donor patient should be approached for risk assessment. Occupational exposures often happen in high-pressure situations and the index patient may be ill, injured, distressed or in pain, undergoing invasive procedures or investigations, or immediately post-operative. Ideally, a doctor known to the patient should make the approach. In most cases the risk assessment will be followed by HIV testing, but the risk

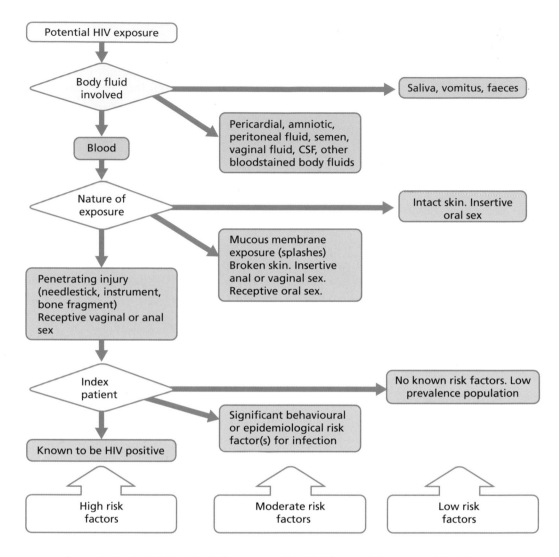

Assess the body fluid involved, the nature of the incident and the status of the donor patient and classify each as high, moderate or low risk. Box 8.7 gives an indication of the need for PEP in line with current guidelines

Figure 8.6
Assessment of exposure to HIV

assessment alone may be helpful in deciding whether to initiate PEP. When approaching the patient, consider the following:

- The patient may be distressed to know that a health worker has been injured
- If the patient **is** at risk of BBV infection, then the prospect of a positive diagnosis has massive implications for the patient
- The duty of care to the patient is unchanged by what has happened. As far as is practicable, the patient is entitled to the same standard of pre-test discussion as if they had requested BBV testing

Box 8.7: Use of post exposure prophylaxis (PEP) after potential exposure to HIV

(Number of high, moderate and low risk factors on assessment of the incident – Fig. 8.6)

High risk	Moderate risk	Low risk	Action
3			PEP usually indicated
2	1		
1	2		Consider PEP
1 or 2		1 or 2	
	3		
	1 or 2	1 or 2	PEP not usually indicated
		3	PEP not indicated

- The patient is entitled to confidentiality. Pre-test discussion should take place in a private room unless this is physically impossible. Only those immediately responsible for the patient's care need be informed of the test and result.

Points to discuss

Tell the patient that a healthcare worker (HCW) has been exposed to body fluids. It isn't necessary to identify the injured HCW if the patient is unaware of the incident. Explain the concern regarding risk of BBV transmission and if necessary the rationale for PEP. If the nature of the exposure means that the patient is not at risk from the HCW, reassure the patient of this. Ask the patient if they have, or are at risk of, HIV or hepatitis. Assess risk factors according to the age and background of the patient.

- The things we are concerned about are HIV, hepatitis B and hepatitis C. Have you ever had a positive test for any of these viruses?
- Have you ever thought you might be at risk? Ever thought that you should be tested and if so, why?
- These viruses are transmitted through blood to blood contact or sex, so I need to ask you a few questions just to check – OK?
- Have you ever injected drugs or had sex with a partner that has done so?
- Ever had sex with anyone from outside the UK? (or explore sexual contacts at home for those originating from high prevalence areas)
- Any sex with men? (if male)

or

- Any bisexual partners? (if female)
- Ever had a blood transfusion or an operation abroad? (if yes explore when, where and under what circumstances).

If the answers to all these questions are negative, then the patient can be regarded as low risk. In most cases it is appropriate to do a test anyway if the patient consents. An HIV antibody result should be obtained urgently, as this may affect immediate management. Testing (and if necessary further pre-test counselling) for hepatitis B (HBsAg) and hepatitis C can be deferred if necessary, for example to the next working day, as post exposure prophylaxis for hepatitis B is effective for several days after the incident.

Cover the points outlined in the section on HIV testing (Ch. 9). In these cases you should usually also:

- discuss what the test is for and establish consent for testing. If in doubt about validity of consent, discuss with the consultant responsible for patient
- ask for the patient's consent to disclose the result to the injured HCW
- make arrangements for the patient to receive the result as soon as it is available.

Follow-up

Those potentially exposed to BBV should be given advice on the risk of onward transmission, whether or not PEP is given. Follow-up testing for HIV and HBsAg at 3 months and hepatitis C at 6 months should be arranged. In those prescribed PEP for HIV, intensive support may be required to manage side effects and continue therapy for 4 weeks. HIV seroconversion may be delayed in those given PEP, so HIV antibody testing should be repeated 6 months after exposure in these cases.

Further Reading

Bennett R, Erin CA, eds. HIV and AIDS testing, screening and confidentiality. Oxford; Oxford University Press: 1999.

Gitlin M. Hepatitis B diagnosis, prevention and treatment. Clin Chem 1997; 43: 1500–1506.

HIV post-exposure prophylaxis: Guidance from the UK Chief Medical Officer's expert advisory group on AIDS. UK Health Departments; July 2000.

Hoofnagle J. Hepatitis C: the clinical spectrum of disease. Hepatology 1997; 26 (S1): 15S–20S (and associated articles).

Lauer GM, Walker BD. Hepatitis C virus infection. N Engl J Med 2001; 345: 41–50.

Lemon SM. Type A viral hepatitis: epidemiology, diagnosis and prevention. Clin Chem 1997; 43: 1494–1499.

US Public Health Service. Updated US public health service guidelines for the management of occupational exposures to HBV, HCV and HIV and recommendations for postexposure prophylaxis. MMWR Morb Mortal Wkly Rep 2001; 50: 1–52.

SELF-ASSESSMENT

You are telephoned by a charge nurse in the accident and emergency department. Jackie (27 years) is an ambulancewoman. She has sustained a needlestick injury while attending to a 40-year-old man who has been injured in a road-traffic accident. His male partner is with him and is not injured. He is conscious and stable in the A+E department.

Questions
a) What do you need to know about the incident?
b) What two facts do you need to know about her from the point of BBV prophylaxis?
c) On the little you know so far, following Figure 8.6, is PEP for HIV likely to be indicated in this case?
d) The incident occurred an hour ago. What are the options?
e) You approach the index patient and his partner. He is unaware of the incident. What do you need to know?
f) If he knows his HIV status to be positive, what additional information do you need?

Answers
a) When did it happen? What sort of needle – an intravenous cannula for resuscitation or an intramuscular needle for sedation or analgesia? What type of injury: superficial scratch or deep intramuscular stab? Was she wearing gloves?
b) What is her hepatitis B vaccination status? Is she, or might she be pregnant?
c) The body fluid is blood – high risk. The injury is a penetrating needlestick – high risk. It is therefore reasonable to recommend PEP for HIV regardless of any risk factors in the index case. This decision will be influenced by the population seroprevalence in the area. The prevalence of HIV infection in homosexual men in the UK (in GUM clinic attendees) is about 15% in London, 2.5% elsewhere; this corresponds to around 10 × the prevalence in heterosexual men.
d) She could commence antiretroviral therapy immediately after a discussion about side effects. If he consents to testing for HIV infection, she could discontinue therapy if his test proves negative. She could defer therapy until his HIV status is known, but the benefit of antiretroviral therapy is likely to be reduced by delay. He may decline testing. She could decide against taking therapy in any case.
e) Does he know his HIV status? Has he ever been tested? If so, when was the last time and what was the result? Would he be prepared to have a test now? What are the implications for him and his partner? Does he know his hepatitis B status? Has he ever been vaccinated?
f) Whether he is taking, or has taken antiretroviral therapy. His current drug therapy and treatment history, and/or his treatment centre and the name of the doctor responsible for his care. This information could be used to modify the PEP regimen given to Jackie, in an attempt to overcome drug resistance in any transmitted virus.

HIV testing, diagnosis and outpatient management

BACKGROUND

HIV is diagnosed in people in the asymptomatic phase of infection, with seroconversion illness or with minor symptoms of HIV. Others, particularly those with heterosexually acquired infection in the UK, may remain undiagnosed until immunosuppression is advanced. The latter group may present with one or more of the opportunistic infections and other conditions diagnostic of AIDS (see Box 9.1). People presenting for screening or treatment of sexually transmitted infection should routinely be offered HIV testing. The testing procedure is described later in this chapter.

From the introduction of highly active antiretroviral therapy (HAART) in the UK from 1995, the number of deaths from AIDS had fallen by around two-thirds by 1999. The number of AIDS cases in the same period fell by over half. Unfortunately, the number of people diagnosed with HIV only when presenting with opportunistic or other infections diagnostic of AIDS remained virtually unchanged and hence the majority of new AIDS cases in the UK occur within 3 months of HIV diagnosis. The care of people with HIV demands a holistic approach to the many physical, psychological and social aspects of the disease, and the multiple problems secondary to its treatment. HIV infection and AIDS present practical, ethical and scientific problems at every stage (Box 9.2).

ORIGIN AND EPIDEMIOLOGY OF HIV/AIDS

The acquired immune deficiency syndrome (AIDS) was first recognized following an unusual cluster of cases of infection with *Pneumocystis carinii* in young homosexual men in the USA in 1981. The virus now known to cause the syndrome was identified under several names in 1983 and 1984, being named human immunodeficiency virus (HIV) in 1986. Recent evidence suggests that the virus was transmitted to man from chimpanzees and other primates in the first half of the 20th century. There are two main HIV types: HIV 1 and HIV 2, HIV 1 being by far the most common worldwide. HIV 2 is found predominantly in West Africa and has a less aggressive course than HIV 1. In 2001, 40 million people worldwide were living with HIV (Box 9.3), about 5 million died and 3 million were newly infected.

Box 9.1: Classification system for HIV infection and AIDS

CD4 cell category	Clinical category A	Clinical category B	Clinical category C
1. ≥ 500 cells/mm^3	A1	B1	C1
2. 200–499 cells/mm^3	A2	B2	C2
3. < 200 cells/mm^3	A3	B3	C3

Clinical conditions

Category A	Category B	Category C
Asymptomatic	Bacillary angiomatosis	Candidiasis of trachea, lungs or oesophagus
Acute HIV infection	Oropharyngeal candidiasis	Invasive cervical cancer
Persistent generalized lymphadenopathy	Vulvovaginal candidiasis	Coccidiomycosis, disseminated or extrapulmonary
Neoplasia	Cervical intraepithelial neoplasis II or III	Cryptococcosis
	Constitutional symptoms	Cryptosporidiosis, diarrhoea >1 month
	Oral hairy leukoplakia	Cytomegalovirus disease
	Herpes zoster: multidermatomal or multiple episode	HIV encephalopathy
	Idiopathic thrombocytopaenic purpura	Herpes simplex: chronic ulcer >1 month duration or bronchitis, pneumonitis or oesophagitis
	Listeriosis	Histoplasmosis: disseminated or extrapulmonary
	Pelvic inflammatory disease	Isosporiasis >1 month
	Peripheral neuropathy	Kaposi's sarcoma
		Burkitt's lymphoma
		Immunoblastic lymphoma
		Primary lymphoma of brain
		Mycobacterium avium complex
		Mycobacterium tuberculosis
		Pneumocystis carinii pneumonia
		Recurrent pneumonia within a 12-month period
		Progressive multifocal leukoencephalopathy
		Salmonella septicaemia
		Cerebral toxoplasmosis
		HIV wasting syndrome

- All conditions in category C are diagnostic of AIDS if diagnosed in the presence of laboratory evidence of HIV infection. Certain conditions including *Pneumocystis carinii* pneumonia and Kaposi's sarcoma are diagnostic of AIDS in the absence of laboratory evidence of HIV.
- In the USA, a CD4 cell count of <200 cells/mm^3 is diagnostic of AIDS, regardless of the clinical status of the patient. This definition does not apply in the UK or Europe.

HIV is transmitted through sexual contact, blood-to-blood contact (re-use or sharing of contaminated needles, transfusion of infected blood) and vertically from mother to child. In Africa, transmission is predominantly through heterosexual sex; men and women are affected in equal numbers. In South East Asia, where the epidemic is in an earlier phase, it is also driven largely by heterosexual transmission. In the USA and Europe more men

Box 9.2: Aspects of HIV management

Physical	Amelioration of physical symptoms
	Detection and treatment of infections
	Infection prophylaxis
	Surveillance for complications such as neoplasms
	Terminal care
Psychological/psychiatric	Impact of diagnosis
	Effect of chronic illness
	Treatments
	Relationships
	Pre-existing and new psychiatric illness
Social	Relationships
	Employment
	Travel
	Accomodation
	Drug use
	Finances
	Nationality and residency
Sexual and reproductive	Partners and partner notification
	Onward transmission
	Fertility
	Pregnancy
Treatments	Antiretroviral therapy
	Availability
	Adherence
	Treatment fatigue
	Side effects
	Drug interactions
	Nutritional support
	Complementary and alternative therapies

Box 9.3: Number of people living with HIV, 2001

	HIV rate, adults 15–49 (%)	Total cases
Worldwide	1.2	40 000 000
Sub-Saharan Africa	9.0	29 000 000
North Africa and Middle East	0.3	500 000
North and South America	0.5	2 900 000
Western Europe	0.3	550 000
Eastern Europe and Central Asia	0.5	1 000 000
East Asia and Pacific	0.1	1 000 000
South and South East Asia	0.6	5 600 000
Australia and New Zealand	0.1	15 000
United Kingdom	0.1	30 000

(Data from UNAIDS, 2002.)

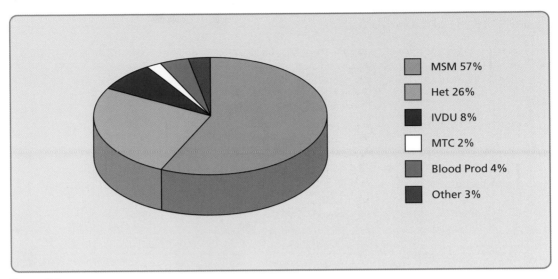

Figure 9.1
Total HIV diagnoses by route of acquisition, UK, to end 2000

than women are infected and the majority of these acquired infection through sex between men. See Figure 9.1 for modes of acquisition in the UK. Intravenous drug use was an important factor in transmission in Scotland, Italy, Spain and Portugal, and continues to contribute to the evolving epidemics in South East Asia and the newly independent states of the former USSR. Healthcare-associated transmission is responsible for large outbreaks of infection in China and has been suggested as an overlooked factor in Africa: its actual contribution to the epidemic is not clear but is probably small. In the UK as in the USA, the number of new diagnoses among heterosexuals overtook those in homosexual men in the late 1990s. Eighty-five per cent of heterosexually acquired infections in the UK are attributable to contact abroad, the majority in Africa, where in some countries the population seroprevalence exceeds 30% (see Fig. 9.2). Of an estimated 42 000 people with HIV in the UK (2001), about one-third are undiagnosed.

PATHOGENESIS AND CLINICAL PRACTICE

HIV attaches to the CD4 receptor borne by a subset of T-helper lymphocytes as well as monocytes, macrophages, dendritic cells and some supporting cells of the nervous system.

HIV belongs to a subgroup of retroviruses called lentiviruses, having the capacity to infect resting (non-multiplying) cells and supporting cells of the central nervous system. As a retrovirus, it possesses the enzyme reverse transcriptase, allowing it to transcribe a DNA copy of its own RNA genome, which when incorporated into host cell DNA results in persisting infection. These features have so far prevented the eradication of HIV by antiretroviral drugs.

Sexual transmission of HIV involves attachment of the virus to mucosal dendritic cells bearing CD4 receptors. Dendritic cells (a form of antigen presenting cell) transport HIV to regional lymph nodes where CD4 bearing lymphocytes are infected. Administering

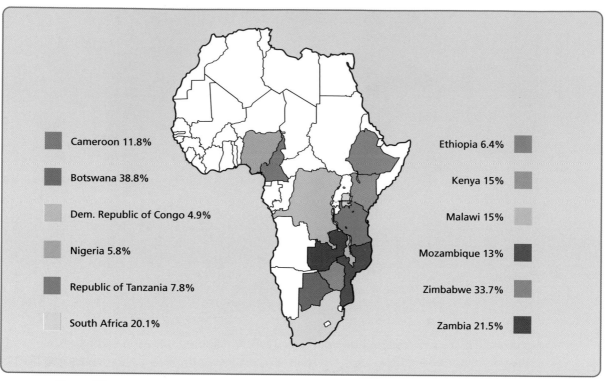

Cameroon 11.8%

Botswana 38.8%

Dem. Republic of Congo 4.9%

Nigeria 5.8%

Republic of Tanzania 7.8%

South Africa 20.1%

Ethiopia 6.4%

Kenya 15%

Malawi 15%

Mozambique 13%

Zimbabwe 33.7%

Zambia 21.5%

Figure 9.2
Estimated seroprevalence in adults aged 15–49 yrs in the twelve most populous nations in sub-Saharan Africa
(Data from UNAIDS, 2002.)

antiretroviral drugs at this stage (ideally within the first hour after infection) may avert the infection and is known as post exposure prophylaxis (PEP).

In the weeks following infection, an initial rapid burst of replication occurs when the plasma viraemia, reflected in the quantitative PCR for HIV viral RNA (the viral load) can reach millions of copies per millilitre. This viraemic phase may be symptomatic (seroconversion illness). The severity of seroconversion illness and the peak of this viraemic phase are indicative of the likely rate of immune deterioration.

The immune system responds to HIV infection as to any other viral infection, mounting a vigorous immune response. This reduces the level of viral replication and the HIV viral load falls in the weeks following seroconversion to a 'set point'. The immune system can control viraemia to a large extent but will not eradicate HIV present as integrated proviral DNA in resting T-cells and macrophages, which do not express viral epitopes on their surface. The immune response involves effector cells including natural killer cells and cytotoxic CD8 T-cells, co-ordinated by CD4 T-helper cells that specifically recognize HIV. However, HIV-specific activated CD4 cells are preferentially infected by HIV and destroyed, so the specific immune response to HIV is depleted in the first few months following infection. The extent to which this specific immune response to HIV is depleted determines the viral set point, which is a major determinant of the rate of immune deterioration (Fig. 9.3).

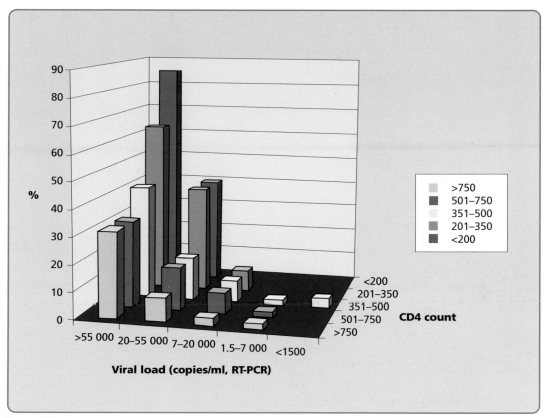

Figure 9.3
Likelihood of developing AIDS within 3 years
(Adapted from Mellors et al, 1997, with permission from American College of Physicians.)

PRIMARY HIV INFECTION

CLINICAL FEATURES

Symptomatic primary HIV infection (also called acute seroconversion illness) occurs in 50–90% of those who acquire HIV. It varies from a mild flu-like syndrome to severe multi-system illness. It occurs 5 days to 4 weeks after HIV acquisition, and lasts for a few days to several weeks. Seroconversion is rarely recognized except in patients who are aware that they have been at risk of HIV infection and who present to someone familiar with the syndrome. There is evidence that treatment at the time of primary HIV infection with highly active antiretroviral therapy (HAART) may affect the long-term prognosis, so the recognition of the syndrome has assumed more importance.

History

Making the diagnosis depends on a high level of suspicion. The patient may be aware of risk, such as unprotected sex with a known HIV+ve partner, within the previous 4 weeks.

Take a full sexual history and explore other risks, particularly injecting drug use. Fever and rash (Fig. 9.4) together have been found to be the strongest predictor of the diagnosis. Clinical features include:

- Fever and fatigue with or without rash (usually maculopapular) and lymphadenopathy
- Oral ulcers and sore throat
- Odynophagia due to oesophageal ulceration or occasionally oesophageal candidiasis. Nausea, vomiting, anorexia and weight loss are less common
- Myalgia, arthralgia, other neurological syndromes and opportunistic infections may complicate the illness.

Examination

Mild pyrexia in over 75%.

Skin. Macular or maculopapular skin rash usually affecting the trunk and head but also the palms of the hands and soles of the feet. The rash may be mistaken for a drug rash, measles, or secondary syphilis. Urticarial or other atypical rash may also be seen.

Mouth. Ulceration, rarely candidiasis.

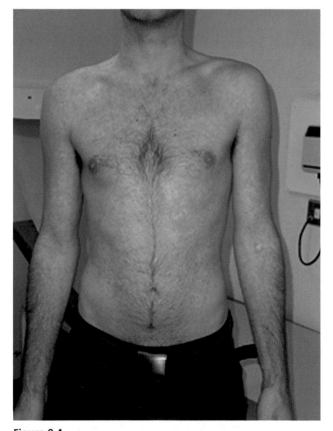

Figure 9.4
Maculopapular rash of HIV seroconversion

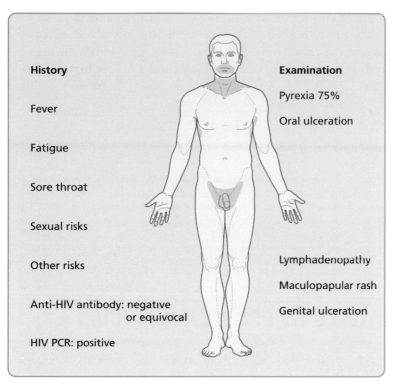

History

Fever

Fatigue

Sore throat

Sexual risks

Other risks

Anti-HIV antibody: negative
          or equivocal

HIV PCR: positive

Examination

Pyrexia 75%

Oral ulceration

Lymphadenopathy

Maculopapular rash

Genital ulceration

Examination Box 9.1 Clinical notes: Primary HIV infection

Lymph nodes. Cervical, axillary and inguinal lymphadenopathy in the second week of the illness.

INVESTIGATION

The diagnosis is confirmed by evidence of HIV viraemia with an incomplete antibody response. HIV antibody tests may be equivocal or negative, although modern EIA tests are sensitive even in early infection. PCR for HIV (viral load) is positive, but false positives occasionally occur. Tests for HIV p24 antigen are less expensive but less sensitive than viral load. An immunoblot or Western blot, if performed, may show the development of antibodies to some HIV antigens but not others. Full blood count may show a lymphopaenia or lymphocytosis, with atypical lymphocytes in up to 50%.

MANAGEMENT

There is evidence that treatment with antiretroviral drugs during seroconversion (or in the first few months after infection) protects the HIV-specific cellular immune response. In some cases this response appears to control HIV viraemia after discontinuation of antiretrovirals. At the time of writing this treatment should ideally be offered through a clinical trial. In patients with a recent history suggesting seroconversion, but a positive EIA and Western blot, a 'detuned' assay has been used. This is a less sensitive form of the standard EIA that fails to detect the low antibody levels seen in recent infection, but does pick up the high levels in established infection. A combination of a positive standard with a negative detuned assay suggests recent seroconversion. Individuals during seroconversion are highly infectious because the viral load is very high. The possibility of further onward transmission, including vertical transmission is greatest at this time, so advice on safer sex and needle sharing should be given

---

Case History

Matthew (27 years) presented to a GUM clinic with a slightly scaly maculopapular rash on his trunk, arms and face. He had had a sore throat and aching muscles the previous week, felt generally unwell and was having night sweats and fevers. He was worried about syphilis having seen publicity regarding a syphilis outbreak. He had had unprotected receptive anal sex several times with the same partner over the course of a weekend, 3 weeks previously. On examination he had cervical and axillary lymphadenopathy. PCR for HIV viral RNA was positive. Syphilis serology was negative. Western blot was positive for p24 antigen with faint bands for p120 and p160 and was reported as equivocal. After detailed discussion he commenced antiretroviral therapy.

THE OUTPATIENT CARE OF PEOPLE WITH HIV

NEWLY DIAGNOSED PATIENT

Giving the diagnosis

Some patients will have been prepared for the diagnosis during a pre-test discussion. However, in patients not considered to be at high risk of infection, discussion may have been brief and the diagnosis may come as a surprise. Similarly, those diagnosed as a result of antenatal testing or the screening of donated blood may be unprepared. Some patients may be able only to express grief or shock and take in little information. Others are better able to discuss prognosis, investigation and treatments. Cover, as a minimum:

- Coping in the immediate future: today and tomorrow
- Who to tell immediately
- The need for outside support
- Arrangement for follow-up or referral
- Who to contact in an emergency.

In the patient who is unprepared for the diagnosis, this may be as much as can be covered in a first meeting. Health advisers, counsellors and other sources of support, such as voluntary agencies should be introduced at this stage, but avoid overwhelming the patient with too many well-meaning people.

If the patient is able to discuss the diagnosis, explore immediate concerns. These often include the fear of death or illness, implications for current and past sexual partners, existing children and future pregnancies, employment and finances, concerns about treatment, or implications for travel, residency or visa applications. It may be possible to determine a history of seroconversion illness, or a previous negative HIV test, to establish whether particular partners or children are at risk. Serum samples previously taken, for example for syphilis serology in pregnancy, may be available from storage for testing. Notification of current and past partners may be tackled immediately or deferred, depending on the risk and the patient's reaction. Discuss the diagnosis in the context of the patient's concerns. Many of the factors placing people at risk of having HIV in a developed nation such as the UK (for example, economic migration from a developing nation, intravenous drug use or homosexuality) may precipitate other practical social problems of more immediate consequence to the patient than the HIV diagnosis. Consider potential psychosocial influences on the patient's response to the diagnosis and treatment (Box 9.4). To patients entitled to receive antiretrovirals where such therapies are freely available, it's appropriate to be optimistic about prognosis in asymptomatic patients, even without knowing the patient's immune status.

Box 9.4: Interaction between psychosocial factors and HIV diagnosis and management

Group	Examples	Potential or feared effect of/on HIV diagnosis
Practical	Financial	Poverty. Inability to serve existing debts. Welfare benefit entitlement (or lack of)
	Employment	Lack of employment security. No sick leave entitlement to attend appointments. Concern about disclosing diagnosis to employer (esp. sex industry work, work in health care)
	Housing	Lack of housing. Inadequate housing. Loss of tenancy or shared housing through disclosure of HIV status
Social	Drug use	Failure (or improvement in) drug supply. Disclosure of use to medical services. Equipment/needle sharing. Violence
	Ethnic group	Isolation. Language difficulties
Relationships	Partner	Risk to sexual partner. Ex-partners. Fear of disclosure. Domestic violence
	Children	Caring for children. Risk of infection in children. Loss of custody
	Family	Rejection. Becoming a burden
Cultural	Community	Fear of disclosure. (Low) priority of own needs
	Spiritual	Acceptance of death. Coping with illness. HIV as punishment
	Health beliefs	Acceptance of and adherence to drug therapy. Non-attendance. Use of complementary and alternative therapies
Fertility	Current pregnancy	Need for termination. HIV transmission. Guilt feelings. Postnatal depression
	Future pregnancies	Avoidance of transmission to serodiscordant partner
Legal	Residency	Entitlement to care. Antiretroviral availability
	Asylum	HIV diagnosis and asylum process
	Culpability	Implications of knowing HIV status on possible transmission to others
Psychological and psychiatric		Exacerbation of previous problems or illness. Low self-esteem (transmission risk). Adjustment to chronic illness. 'Second life syndrome'. Anger and despair. Suicide risk

INITIAL MEDICAL ASSESSMENT

At the first appointment following diagnosis a full medical history and examination should be performed. In those patients who are clearly unwell with suspected AIDS, the focus may be on acute physical problems (Ch. 11) and a more comprehensive psychosocial assessment is deferred.

History

First address the patient's own agenda. Listening to the story of what led up to the diagnosis of HIV is often a good way to get a feeling for the patient's mental state, knowledge about the disease and background. Record a full medical history (see Clinical notes below). Some patients will be completely asymptomatic, but many will report minor symptoms of HIV infection on specific enquiry. These might include previously unexplained fatigue, fever, weight loss or diarrhoea. Minor skin symptoms such as dryness or scaling of the skin, fungal infections of the skin or nails (*Candida*, seborrhoeic dermatitis, Tinea) are usual, as are bacterial infections such as folliculitis. A past history of troublesome recurrent herpes simplex infection, one or more episodes of zoster (Figs 9.5, 9.6), or episodes of respiratory infection may be recalled. Vaginal or oral candidiasis may have been a problem. In patients with multiple minor symptoms of HIV infection, a careful systemic review is useful to detect symptoms of commoner co-existing disease or opportunistic infection, particularly respiratory symptoms (e.g. *Pneumocystis carinii* pneumonia or tuberculosis) or odynophagia (oesophageal candidiasis). Asking about appetite, weight loss, diarrhoea and neurological symptoms should also be routine. If physical symptoms suggesting an episode of depressive illness are detected, always explore more thoroughly, preferably using a standard depression score as a guide. Perform a full systemic examination, even in asymptomatic patients, paying particular attention to the whole of the skin surface (looking for seborrhoeic dermatitis, Kaposi's

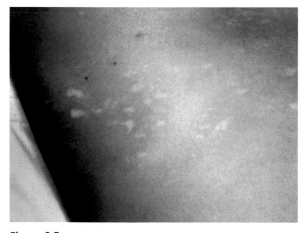

Figure 9.5
Scarring of previous zoster

sarcoma, psoriasis, fungal and bacterial infection) and the oropharynx (*Candida*, gingivitis, oral hairy leukoplakia) (Figs 9.7, 9.8). Routine baseline tests in asymptomatic or minimally symptomatic patients include tests of immune status and serological tests for previous exposure to pathogens causing HIV-related complications. Other tests may be appropriate in patients with specific symptoms (see Ch. 11).

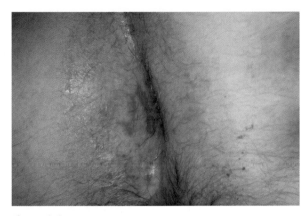

Figure 9.6
Recurrent perianal HSV in a man with HIV infection

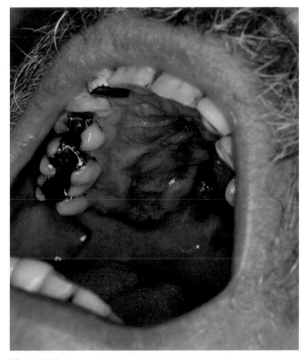

Figure 9.7
Kaposi's sarcoma of the palate

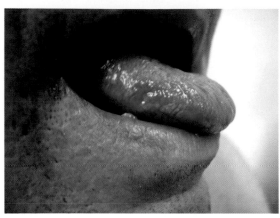

Figure 9.8
Oral hairy leukoplakia and angular cheilitis at HIV diagnosis

Clinical notes: History taking in HIV infection

Symptoms of infection

Weight loss, tiredness, lethargy, night sweats, fevers
Recurrent upper respiratory tract infections, sinusitis
Breathlessness, productive or non-productive cough
Chronic diarrhoea
Chronic, recurrent or treatment resistant vulvovaginal candidiasis
Skin problems: rashes, scaling, itching, nail infections, warts
Mouth ulcers, gingivitis, dental problems

Past medical history

History of possible seroconversion illness (may be helpful in determining partners/children at risk)
History of zoster, particularly multi-episode or multi-dermatomal zoster
Recurrent oral, genital or other herpes simplex virus infections
Severe bacterial infections
Tuberculosis or contact with TB
Hypertension, diabetes, ischaemic heart disease
Mental health
Hepatitis
Gynaecological history
Sexually transmitted infections
Abnormal cervical cytology smears
Registration with a general practitioner

Social history

Relationship status, partners, sexual history (including partners at risk of infection), children (?at risk of infection)
Existing support services and networks (e.g. social work, drugs worker)
Residency, accommodation, employment, income
Smoking, alcohol, recreational drugs
Travel history, previous residency, tropical diseases
Prescription medications
Opiate substitutes, benzodiazepines, dosages, supply arrangements and frequency in current or ex-opiate users
Vaccinations
Contraception

Clinical notes: History taking in HIV infection – (cont'd)

Full systemic review

Checklist: investigations in HIV infection
Confirmatory HIV antibody test (occasional factitious illness, laboratory or labelling error)
Full blood count
Urea and electrolytes
Liver function tests
Hepatitis A serology in MSM, IVDU and those with HCV
Hepatitis B serology according to exposure/vaccination history
Hepatitis C serology (and if risk factors for infection identified and liver function is abnormal, do hepatitis C vRNA if antibody negative)
Toxoplasma IgG
Cytomegalovirus IgG
Epstein–Barr Virus IgG
Syphilis serology
CD4 count
Quantitative PCR for HIV viral RNA ('viral load')
HIV resistance testing

Chest X-ray
Full routine STI screen
Cervical smear in women
Anal smear in homosexual men

Consider:
Pregnancy test
PPD testing
G-6-PD screening in those of Mediterranean, Indian, Asian or African origin

MANAGEMENT

At an early review consultation the results of serological tests and surrogate markers should be available. The CD4 count and HIV viral load are the most reliable surrogate markers of immune status and the likelihood of disease progression and death (Box 9.5). The results of these tests may show considerable sample-to-sample variation due to the margin of laboratory error and biological variability. At least two sets of results from the same laboratory, usually taken two or more weeks apart, should be seen before any firm

Box 9.5: Surrogate markers of HIV infection

Marker	Affected by	Notes on interpretation
CD4 count	Laboratory variation Intercurrent illness Total lymphocyte count	Normal range 500–1500 cells/mm^3 A significant drop in CD4 count is regarded as a 30% change in absolute number or 3 percentage points Average decline is 60 cells/mm^3/year CD4 count of 500 cells/mm^3 is equivalent to 29%, 200 cells/mm^3 is 14%
Viral load	Assay used Laboratory variation	A significant change in viral load is 0.5 log$_{10}$ or 3-fold Peak viral load at seroconversion may be >10^{6}copies/ml A 'set point' is established at about 24 weeks after infection which determines the rate of CD4 count decline

conclusions are drawn. Many patients will wish to discuss in detail the prognostic implications of CD4 count and viral load results. Others will prefer simply to be advised what treatment if any, is required. Further management is guided by clinical condition and CD4 count (see Fig. 9.9). Men who have acquired HIV through sex with men tend to be diagnosed earlier than heterosexual men and women. In the UK in the late 1990s, the median CD4 count at the time of diagnosis was around 350 cells/mm^3 in homosexual men compared to 200–250 cells/mm^3 in heterosexual men and women. Asymptomatic patients with CD4 count of >500 cells/mm^3, and many of those with CD4 counts in the range

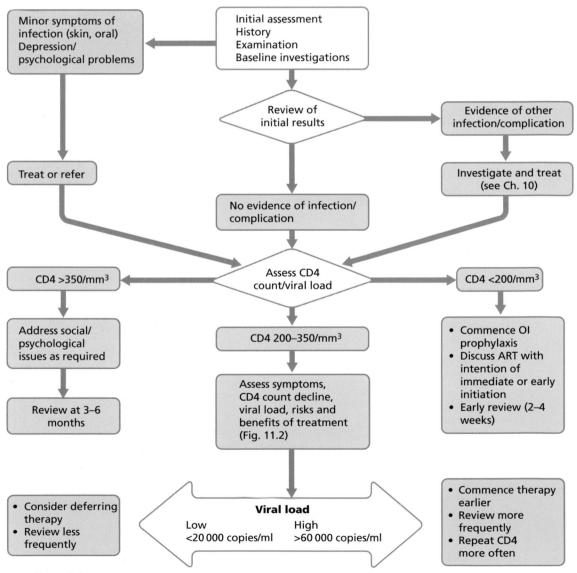

Figure 9.9
Management of people with newly diagnosed HIV infection

200–500 cells/mm^3 can be reviewed 3–6 monthly once immediate social and practical problems have been addressed. Treatment for and advice on minor symptoms of HIV infection may be given (Ch. 10). In patients with CD4 count of <350 cells/mm^3, or with symptoms, it is appropriate to begin discussions in preparation for antiretroviral therapy (Ch. 11). Antiretroviral therapy and/or prophylaxis against opportunistic infection must be considered more immediately if the CD4 count is <200 cells/mm^3. In patients with viral load between 200 and 350 cells/mm^3 the viral load may also influence the decision on when to begin discussions about antiretroviral therapy.

PPD testing

In the UK, routine PPD testing of people with HIV is not universal. If performed, a 5 mm^3 induration at 48 hours after a 5 ml (or 10 mm^3 after 10 ml) intradermal injection of 1:1000 tuberculin is regarded as positive. Patients with reactive tests should be investigated for TB and if no active infection found, receive chemoprophylaxis with isoniazid 300 mg daily for 9 months. Potential problems include reactivity due to prior BCG vaccination, anergy at CD4 counts of <400 cells/mm^3 (becoming more common with lower CD4 count), and the resulting difficulty in interpreting the response. Whether or not skin testing is routinely offered, maintain a high level of vigilance for symptoms of possible TB in patients originating from or travelling to endemic areas, or with other risk factors for TB such as homelessness.

Vaccination

Patients with high CD4 count should be vaccinated early while immunity is intact. If the CD4 count is <200 cells/mm^3 and antiretrovirals are likely to be commenced imminently, it may be preferable to wait until immunity has recovered with HAART before attempting a vaccine course. If vaccines are given at low CD4 counts, they should be repeated once the CD4 count has recovered to 200 cells/mm^3. Most live vaccines are contra-indicated in people with HIV, including oral polio vaccine, BCG, MMR, oral typhoid vaccine and yellow fever. There is some concern that vaccines cause a transient rise in viral load. This may be important in pregnancy (where a rise in viral load may increase the risk of transmission) and in patients with advanced disease. Recommended vaccines include:

Hepatitis vaccination (see Ch. 8). Hepatitis B vaccination is recommended in patients who have no serological evidence of vaccine or exposure induced immunity and who are at continuing risk of hepatitis B. Since in practice the risk factors for HIV infection and hepatitis B exposure coincide in so many cases, it is reasonable to offer vaccination to all HIV positive patients. Patients also at continued risk of hepatitis A infection, particularly those co-infected with hepatitis B or C, should be given combined vaccines.

Pneumococcal vaccine. Polyvalent pneumococcal vaccine is widely regarded as beneficial and is recommended for all patients with HIV, although one randomized controlled trial in Africa showed more cases of pneumonia in vaccinated subjects.

Influenza vaccine. Recommended at high CD4 count with undetectable viral load (although there is no proof of benefit). In advanced disease the marginal effect may be outweighed by the increase in viral load.

Social support

Many larger clinics will have established links to support services, including counsellors, psychologists, social workers and voluntary agencies. Patients should be referred early to agencies providing support with benefits, accommodation, drug use, legal issues, asylum and residency issues as appropriate. In smaller clinics and non-specialist settings, it may be useful to use national organizations for guidance and support. Many patients find it hard to approach such agencies independently, particularly in the stressful period following diagnosis. Giving leaflets, addresses or phone numbers may not be sufficient: an informal referral or personal introduction may be more helpful.

ROUTINE FOLLOW-UP

Most people with HIV in the UK are cared for as outpatients in a hospital based clinic, although the holistic and long-term nature of HIV medicine lends itself well to primary care. Patients should be strongly encouraged to inform their GP of the diagnosis even if the majority of HIV-related care is to be provided by a specialist centre. Patients who remain well without antiretroviral drugs, or who are stable on HAART, are often routinely reviewed at 3 or 6 monthly intervals. A visit for blood taking 2 weeks or so before review allows results to be available for discussion. New physical symptoms, psychological state, changes in personal and social circumstances and current immune status may be discussed. Some patients become hypervigilant in monitoring physical symptoms, particularly as they adjust to the diagnosis. Support and reassurance must be combined with appropriate investigations that can partly be guided by the CD4 count. Physical examination may not be necessary in patients with good immunity and no symptoms, but screening tests for infection and malignancy should be considered regularly (Box 9.6). Review of potential side effects, adherence and additional monitoring tests are important in those taking antiretroviral therapy. Regular testing for sexually transmitted infections has been overlooked in some HIV infected patients in the past. As bacterial and viral STIs may both facilitate HIV transmission and have more severe consequences in HIV infected patients, patients at risk of STI should undergo regular testing. One recognized difficulty experienced by doctors caring for chronically infected HIV patients, is a change in the interpersonal relationship over time, making the type of questions routinely asked in sexual health care feel unacceptably intrusive. It may be easier for a professional who is not closely involved with the patient's HIV care to tackle discussion of and testing for STIs.

Psychological and psychiatric support

The psychological effects of HIV infection range from acute adjustment reactions in response to the initial diagnosis of HIV, to the reaction to the possibility of increased survival with HAART in those who have accepted the prospect of a foreshortened lifespan – the 'second life syndrome'. The frequency of new psychiatric diagnosis is increased compared to the general population and the lifetime prevalence of major depression in people with HIV was estimated at 22–56% prior to the availability of HAART. Many units caring for those with HIV have formal links with psychological and

Box 9.6: Routine follow-up procedures in HIV outpatient care

Procedure	Frequency	Indication, rationale
Physical examination	Annually	Detection of painless conditions such as Kaposi's sarcoma
Ophthalmology review	6 monthly	All patients with CD4 count of <50 cells/mm^3 (Risk of CMV retinitis)
Lipid profile Blood pressure Cardiovascular risk factors	Annually (increase frequency if abnormal)	Lipid abnormalities in people taking HAART
CD4 count Viral load	3–6 monthly	Monitoring of disease progression
Full blood count Clinical chemistry Liver function tests	3–6 monthly	Anaemia, thrombocytopaenia common with HIV infection and HAART Hepatotoxicity common with HAART (abnormal LFTs in 8–20%)
Cervical smear or colposcopic examination	Annually	Increased risk of CIN and possibly carcinoma
Anal cytology smear	Annually in all homosexual men	Increased risk of anal carcinoma Some evidence that routine screening is cost-effective
Influenza vaccination	Annually in October	Complications of influenza such as bacterial pneumonia more common in HIV (though no proof of benefit)
Syphilis serology Screening for bacterial STIs	Offer annually to all patients. 3–6 monthly in patients with multiple partners/change of partner	STIs may have more serious sequelae in HIV and increase the risk of transmission

psychiatric services making referral straightforward. If the patient's well-being, personal circumstances and concerns are the focus of each review appointment, rather than surrogate marker results, the opportunity to detect psychological and psychiatric morbidity is increased. The wide range of disorders encountered cannot be covered here, but the ability to assess patients with possible depression is particularly useful. Mirtazapine and sertraline are well tolerated and do not interact with licensed antiretrovirals.

DECISIONS BASED ON CD4 COUNT AND VIRAL LOAD

Large cohort studies show that certain markers of HIV infection, termed surrogate markers, are closely associated with the likelihood of development of AIDS and death. A smaller number of randomized controlled trials of antiretroviral therapy have shown that the rise in CD4 count and fall in viral load that occurs with treatment is associated with a reduction in the rate of opportunistic infection and death – termed clinical endpoints. The outcomes of the overwhelming majority of randomized controlled trials of HIV therapy in

- Depressed mood
- Loss of interest and enjoyment
- Reduced energy
- Reduced concentration and attention
- Reduced self-esteem and self-confidence
- Ideas of guilt and unworthiness
- Bleak and pessimistic views of the future
- Ideas or acts of self-harm or suicide
- Disturbed sleep
- Diminished appetite

recent years have been measured in terms of surrogate markers only, rather than clinical endpoints. The CD4 count and viral load, the most widely used surrogate markers, provide in combination the best currently available prediction of the likelihood of disease progression and of treatment effect. Interpretation of, and particularly comparisons between, studies of different interventions using these markers are limited by their incomplete ability to reflect clinical outcomes. Other surrogate markers including CD4/8 ratio, b2 microglobulin, and p24 antigen are no longer used in routine clinical practice.

CD4 COUNT

The CD4 count is a measure of the extent of damage to the immune system reflected in depletion of the T-helper lymphocyte subset bearing the CD4 surface antigen. It is the most reliable single predictor of the immediate probability of developing opportunistic infection, AIDS or death. The degree of immunosuppression influences the differential diagnosis in a patient presenting with, for example, respiratory symptoms, the need for antiretroviral therapy and the commencement and discontinuation of opportunistic infection prophylaxis. Increases in CD4 with treatment provide an imperfect reflection (probably an underestimate) of the clinical benefit of antiretroviral therapy. Patients who are not taking therapy and with CD4 counts of <200 cells/mm^3 may be seen more frequently, and monthly visits are sometimes appropriate in patients with a CD4 count less than 50 cells/mm^3.

VIRAL LOAD

Quantitative measurement of HIV RNA 'viral load' is a predictor of future disease progression and death. In the untreated patient, the viral load 'set point' is indicative of the likely rate of decline in CD4 count, so patients with high viral loads may be considered for therapy sooner than those with low viral load, to avoid the possibility of CD4 count falling substantially below 200 cells/mm^3 and the associated risk of opportunistic infection (OI). Viral load is the best marker of response to antiretroviral therapy and reductions in viral load partly predict the clinical response to treatment. Viral load measurement is usually by PCR amplification (RT-PCR) or b-DNA assay: it is important to know which test is used in clinical decision making as RT-PCR gives a consistently higher result. The lower limit of detection for the test may be 400, 50 or occasionally 5 copies per ml of plasma. Commercial viral load assays are designed to quantify subtype B viruses of the main (M) group of HIV 1, predominant in Europe and North America. They may not perform as reliably in infection with other subtypes (A, C–K) of HIV 1, or HIV 2, found in Asia or Africa.

PATIENT INFORMATION

Sharing information with the patient is important at all stages of disease. Immediately after diagnosis the patient may be too shocked or distressed to absorb details. Information in small amounts, repeated if necessary and using appropriate language and level of detail for the patient's intellect and educational background is most useful. Try to ensure that all members of the team are giving information and that it is consistent. Most, but not all patients want detailed information, so it is worth asking directly at an early consultation how much the patient likes to know. Intelligent patients, whatever their educational background, may require medical words and phrases explaining in simple terms at first but very rapidly acquire sophisticated knowledge and understanding. Staying abreast of this developing knowledge and adapting to the level of detail required can be challenging. Expert patients whose knowledge exceeds yours can be a great source of information. Review the patient literature, much of which is excellent, and keep either in the clinic or personally a stock of booklets and leaflets. Patients increasingly access the same sources of information as healthcare staff on the internet, so recommending particular sites to patients (and following up patient recommendations) while keeping track of newly posted information helps to facilitate constructive discussion.

Checklist: sources of information

- www.aidsmap.com
- www.aidsinfo.nih.gov
- www.natap.org
- www.i-base.org.uk
- THT Direct Phoneline 0845 1221 200
- i-Base Treatment Phoneline 0808 8006013

HIV TESTING AND PRE-TEST DISCUSSION

BACKGROUND

Pre- and post-test discussion around HIV antibody testing is an important component of routine sexual health care wherever it is delivered. The procedure, also termed voluntary counselling and testing (VCT), is regarded as a vital component in HIV prevention efforts worldwide, with benefits applicable in both high and low income nations. Family or general practitioners, having a detailed knowledge of a patient and their personal circumstances, may be the most appropriate people to undertake pre-test discussion and testing for HIV. However, although the stigma attached to testing has reduced in recent years, many people choose to undergo testing with the anonymity offered by GUM clinics in the UK. Others may be diagnosed as part of the investigation of clinical symptoms, for insurance purposes, or as a result of partner notification or blood donation. An 'opt-out' policy of universal antenatal testing for HIV applies in many states in the USA and parts of Europe. Consequently, women may be first diagnosed during pregnancy. The prognosis of HIV infection has improved dramatically in countries where HAART is available, but even here the impact of a positive diagnosis on the individual is only marginally diminished.

Diagnostic tests

The most widely used screening tests are enzyme immunoassays performed on serum, confirmed if positive by a supplementary test such as a Western blot. See Box 9.7 for details of tests used.

PRE-TEST DISCUSSION

Full pre- and post-test counselling for HIV testing might include:

- Information on the test and its implications
- Comprehensive risk assessment

Box 9.7: Laboratory tests of HIV infection

Screening tests

Enzyme immunoassay (EIA)	Test for specific antibody against the virus Negative in the first few days of seroconversion Sensitivity and specificity >99% Ability to detect anti-HIV 2 or anti-HIV group O dependent on type of test – establish the test used by your lab Fourth generation EIA detects p24 antigen as well as antibody
Rapid tests	EIA or latex agglutination tests providing results in about 10 mins. High sensitivity and specificity but usually confirmed by standard tests. Can be used in STI clinics, or obstetric departments with high prevalence populations
Saliva tests 'Detuned assay'	Comparable sensitivity and specificity to serum tests A low sensitivity EIA may be used in combination with a conventional assay to determine whether HIV infection is recently acquired, for epidemiological estimates of incidence, or for diagnosis of recent infection

Confirmatory tests

Western blot or immunoblot	HIV proteins bound to nitrocellulose strips to which HIV antibodies bind Antibodies to two of p24, gp41, and gp120/160 are diagnostic. Indeterminate results may indicate seroconversion
HIV RNA or DNA detection	Polymerase chain reaction or branched DNA (bDNA) assays detect and quantify HIV RNA: 'viral load' tests. Used to confirm infection when screening tests are equivocal, and as a surrogate marker. Lower limit of detection usually 400 or 50 copies/ml, but 5 copies/ml is available
HIV p24 antigen	Detection of p24 antigen by EIA is useful in the diagnosis of primary HIV infection and as a surrogate marker of disease progression where HIV RNA detection is unavailable

- Informed consent
- Preparation for test outcome: effect on health, life expectancy, sexual and emotional relationships, existing children and future procreation, treatment, psychological impact, sources of support, visas, travel and residency
- Post-test counselling, giving support and follow-up to those with positive results, attempting to promote behaviour change in those with negative results.

Discussion is probably a better description than counselling for the procedure usually undertaken. If HIV testing is routinely offered to all individuals requesting tests for sexually transmitted diseases, pre-test discussion must in most cases be brief. Where the majority of those requesting a test have a low probability of being infected, it is not practical to cover all of the above points in detail in every case. In this situation the most important component of the discussion is a comprehensive risk assessment. This allows a 'two-tier' system, testing of the majority of individuals after a basic discussion, but identifying those at significant risk of infection and offering more intensive discussion, and support including some or all of the aspects described above. Where the population seroprevalence is higher, a two-tier system may not be appropriate. An efficient but sensitive discussion prior to undertaking a test should allow sufficient information to be given to the patient, allowing informed consent to be given without making discussion cursory. The following is loosely based on the UK Department of Health guidelines.

Reason for testing

Establish the reason for requesting a test, the understanding of the difference between HIV infection and AIDS and the patient's own perception of HIV risk.

Risk of infection

Assess the patient's risk of HIV infection. As a minimum, consider:

1. Sexual risks. A routine sexual history may well have been taken as part of a routine consultation (see Ch. 1). Concentrate on known overall risk; in the assessment of lifetime risk it is unlikely to be helpful to explore the potential HIV risk of several different sexual partners. It may be relevant to ask about:
   a) Peno-vaginal or peno-anal sex without a condom with partners known to have HIV
   b) Peno-vaginal or peno-anal sex without a condom with partners (especially regular) from or in areas of high HIV prevalence (see Box 9.3)
   c) Men having sex with men. Without exception all men must be asked about history of sex with other men:
      - unprotected anal sex with partners of known HIV seropositive status, or partners of unknown status
      - oral sex without a condom with partners of known HIV seropositive status
      - oral sex without a condom with multiple partners
      - sex in places with high HIV seroprevalence among MSM.
2. Intravenous drug use or sex with current or ex-intravenous drug users. Explore needle sharing in these cases.
3. Tattoos undertaken in non-professional (e.g. prison) settings.

4. Exposure to blood products including blood donation (safe in Europe and USA from 1991).
5. Occupational risk (nurses, doctors, dentists, emergency services).

If any of the above points elicit a potentially significant risk, a more detailed discussion prior to testing may be appropriate. In some clinics this is done by specialist counsellors or health advisers.

Advantages and disadvantages of testing

Discuss the advantages or disadvantages of doing the test. Patients who have requested a test may regard these as self-evident and may not wish to explore this point. In the individual with no identifiable risk factors for infection in a low prevalence population, it may be sufficient to confirm that the patient is prepared to deal with the unlikely outcome of a positive result, and that now is a good time to be tested. In others, potential advantages to be discussed include:

- Protection of current or future sexual partners and the prevention of vertical transmission
- Access to preventative and therapeutic care including antiretroviral drugs where available
- Allows life decisions to be made
- Resolves anxiety, especially in those at low risk.

Potential disadvantages include:

- Psychological impact of dealing with a diagnosis
- Social stigma and impact on relationships
- Employment and financial implications.

It is worth identifying someone whom the patient may confide in for initial support in the event of a positive result. Patients' concerns about a possible HIV diagnosis and its implications differ with culture and social and ethnic background. The pros and cons of testing are different depending upon circumstance. For example, living with a diagnosis of HIV from the perspective of an African national with a UK student visa may not include the possibility of long-term antiretroviral treatment.

The window period

Explain the limitations of the test, including the fact that the test for HIV antibody has a 'window period' of 3 months. Make it explicitly clear that this means that seroconversion for HIV antibody may not occur until up to three months after acquisition of the virus. It may be appropriate to defer or repeat the test.

Confidentiality

Outline the extent and limits of confidentiality in the system within which testing is done, including contact with other agencies, insurance companies and legal bodies. In the UK, life insurance companies do not ask questions about negative tests for HIV infection but other insurance companies may do so. General practitioners are advised by the British Medical Association not to answer 'lifestyle' type questions about patients.

Further Reading

American Psychiatric Association Practice Guidelines. Practice Guidelines for the treatment of patients with HIV/AIDS. Am J Psychiatry 2000; suppl 157: 11.

Anderson JMD (ed). A guide to the clinical care of women with HIV. Washington: HRSA. Available at http://www.hrsa.gov/hab

Apoola A, Ahmad S, Radcliffe K. Primary HIV infection. Int Jour STD & AIDS 2002; 13: 71–78.

Ho DD, Neumann AU, Perelson AS, Chen W, Leonard JM, Markowitz M. Rapid turnover of plasma virions and CD4 lymphocytes in HIV-1 infection. Nature 1995; 373: 123–126.

Johnson RP. The dynamics of T-lymphocyte turnover in AIDS. AIDS 2000; 14: S3–S9.

Mellors JW, Munoz A, Giorgi JV. Plasma viral load and CD4+ lymphocytes as prognostic markers of HIV-1 infection. Ann Intern Med 1997; 126(12): P946–954.

Mortimer J, McHenry A, Evans B. HIV and AIDS in the UK - an epidemiological review at the year 2000. In: Gazzard BG, Johnson M, Miles A (eds). The effective management of HIV/AIDS. London; Aesculapius Medical Press: 2001.

Rosenberg ES, Altfield M, Poon SH et al. Immune control of HIV 1 after early treatment of acute infection. Nature 2000; 407: 523–526.

UNAIDS. Report on the global HIV/AIDS epidemic 2002. Geneva; UNAIDS: 2002.

Unlinked Anonymous Surveys Steering Group. Prevalence of HIV and hepatitis infections in the United Kingdom 2001. London; Department of Health: 2002.

SELF-ASSESSMENT

Alfred is a 28-year-old Nigerian PhD student in his first year. He has seen his GP three times in the last 8 weeks for antibiotic treatment of lower respiratory-tract infections. His GP suggested he had an HIV test. He received a positive result a week ago. You see him for the first time in the HIV outpatient clinic.

Questions
a) What medical issues take priority in the history?
b) What psychosocial issues might affect this case?

Answers
a) Assess his current and recent symptoms. Determine whether he has an opportunistic infection which would need immediate investigation. Does he still have respiratory symptoms? Did they resolve completely with antibiotics? If not, explore in detail, discuss breathlessness, cough, sputum and chest pain and consider the possibility of bacterial infection, PCP or TB.
   Any other recent symptoms: Are there other symptoms to suggest immunosuppression? Did he get oral thrush with antibiotics? Any skin changes, weight loss, diarrhoea, neurological symptoms?
   The risk of other problems and infections: When was he last in Nigeria? What previous infectious illnesses has he had? Any vaccinations?
b) His reaction to the diagnosis, whether it was expected and how he has coped since. His previous experience of HIV infection may depend on whether he knows of people diagnosed with HIV in the Northern hemisphere or in Africa. His family and support network – here or elsewhere? He may have a support network in the UK, but is he able to tell them of the diagnosis? Does he have a current regular partner(s)? Regular or ex-partners and children in Nigeria? What is his immigration status – student or other visa. What are his plans after the PhD? Is he financially secure? Does he work to support his PhD and if so has he been well enough to work recently?

Symptomatic HIV infection and AIDS

10

BACKGROUND

Untreated HIV infection almost invariably results in a progressive deterioration in immune function. Following seroconversion (Ch. 9), an asymptomatic or minimally symptomatic phase of 3–8 years usually follows. An AIDS-defining condition will supervene on average 8–11 years after seroconversion in people who do not receive antiretroviral therapy (Fig. 10.1). A small minority of people will remain asymptomatic, with well-preserved immune function for 20 years or more without treatment. In the

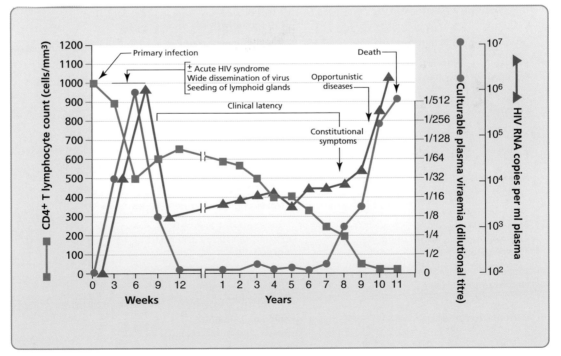

Figure 10.1
The typical course of untreated HIV infection as understood in the early 1990s. It was later appreciated that HIV replication continues throughout the period of clinical latency, the number of HIV RNA copies per ml plasma during this period being 10^3–10^6 copies/ml
(From Fauci et al, 1996, with permission from American College of Physicians.)

majority, however, progressive defects in T-cell, B-cell, cytotoxic and natural-killer cell mediated defences render the individual susceptible to a variety of infections and other complications. Opportunistic infections (OI) are those due to pathogens causing asymptomatic infection or minor illness in the immunocompetent but potentially life-threatening systemic infection or malignancy in those with immunosuppression. Many of the problems affecting those with HIV are caused by organisms that are pathogenic in those without immunosuppression (such as herpes viruses and TB), but which cause more extensive, severe or atypical disease in HIV infection (see Box 10.1). In high-income and some middle-income nations (e.g. Brazil), the availability of highly active antiretroviral

---

Box 10.1: Opportunistic pathogens in HIV/AIDS

Pathogen	Disease in HIV infection
Bacteria	
Skin pathogens	
Staphylococcus aureus	Abscesses, furuncles
Respiratory pathogens	
Streptococcus pneumoniae	Pneumonia
Haemophilus influenzae	
Enteric pathogens	
Salmonella, Shigella, Campylobacter spp.	Gastroenteritis, septicaemia
Mycobacterium tuberculosis	Pulmonary TB
	Non-pulmonary TB
Mycobacterium avium complex	Usually disseminated disease
Fungi	
Pneumocystis carinii	Pneumonia
	Retinitis
Candida spp.	Oropharyngeal candidiasis
	Vulvovaginal candidiasis
	Oesophageal candidiasis
Cryptococcus neoformans	Meningitis
Histoplasma capsulatum	Respiratory symptoms
	TB-like illness
	(Travel/origin in southern states of USA)
Protozoans	
Cryptosporidium, Microsporidium	Chronic diarrhoea and wasting
Toxoplasma gondii	Encephalitis
Viruses	
Herpes simplex 1 and 2	Oral, genital lesions
	Encephalitis
Varicella-zoster virus	Shingles
	Zoster ophthalmicus
Cytomegalovirus (CMV)	Retinitis
	Encephalitis
	Oesophagitis and colitis
	Adrenitis (adrenal failure in late-stage HIV)
JC virus	Progressive multifocal leukoencephalopathy

therapy (HAART) reduced the incidence of such opportunistic infections by up to 80% between 1995 and 1999. Some OIs respond to treatment with HAART alone (cytomegalovirus disease, Kaposi's sarcoma, *Cryptosporidium*) and survival after first-episode infection and with other HIV-related complications such as progressive multifocal leukoencephalopathy (PML) has also improved. Modern HIV care involves the treatment of multi-system disease, prophylaxis against opportunistic infections, initiation and maintenance of antiretroviral therapy (where available) and the management of the resultant polypharmacy. In people with mild-to-moderate immunosuppression, the relief of symptoms of minor conditions is combined with routine monitoring and alertness to the development of less common, but more serious complications. The range and severity of infections and the probability of malignancy is inversely related to CD4 count. The problems encountered as immunity deteriorates can be considered in five partly overlapping groups:

- Conditions due to HIV infection
- Increased susceptibility to common community acquired infections
- Susceptibility to newly-acquired opportunistic infections
- Reactivation of quiescent infections
- Malignancies.

When the CD4 count is over 350 cells/mm³ patients are often asymptomatic, although constitutional symptoms of HIV or minor opportunistic infections may require treatment. Opportunistic infections diagnostic of AIDS are usually seen at CD4 count less than 200 cells/mm³ and rarely at CD4 count over 500 cells/mm³ (see Box 9.1). Certain AIDS indicator diseases are seen irrespective of CD4 count and include TB, Kaposi's sarcoma and non-Hodgkins lymphoma, but these too are more common at lower CD4 counts.

PATHOGENESIS AND CLINICAL PRACTICE

The untreated natural history of immune deterioration due to HIV is variable, affected by factors including host genetics and age but probably not gender or intravenous drug use. Following seroconversion (Ch. 9), HIV viral load is said to reach a 'set point'. Variables thought to determine this set point include viral factors and host genetic factors including HLA subtype and other variations in cell surface markers. The 'set point' in fact increases gradually over the years in untreated infection. The HIV-specific immune response persisting after seroconversion is partly mediated by CD8 cytotoxic lymphocytes (CTL), central to the control of viral infections. In some people, CTL recognizing a wide range of HIV epitopes are preserved and viraemia is well controlled. These individuals have low (sometimes undetectable) viral load and CD4 depletion occurs slowly or not at all. Such individuals are termed slow progressors or long-term non-progressors.

In the majority of people, immune control of HIV is incomplete and active viral replication continues. Massive numbers of short-lived virions are produced each day. These virions induce the destruction of large numbers of CD4 cells, the minority by direct infection. The majority of CD4 cell destruction appears to be by apoptosis, autoimmune killing or other processes affecting cells not infected with HIV. Memory CD4 T-helper cells specific for infections to which the individual has previously been exposed or vaccinated, for example, mycobacteria and herpes viruses, as well as naïve CD4 cells are gradually depleted over the course of several years. These changes parallel other immune defects rendering the individual susceptible to new infections, the re-activation of quiescent infection and the development of malignancies, often initiated by viral cofactors.

MINOR SYMPTOMS OF HIV INFECTION

Constitutional symptoms and minor opportunistic infections can affect quality of life at all stages of disease. Common problems include diseases of the skin and oral cavity. If recognized as manifestations of HIV infection in undiagnosed patients presenting to medical services, they may prompt HIV testing. At a CD4 count of 350–500 cells/mm^3 symptoms are usually tolerable or relieved by specific treatment. As the CD4 count declines, such symptoms may become more troublesome. If they are difficult to manage symptomatically this can influence the decision to initiate antiretroviral therapy sooner rather than later.

CONSTITUTIONAL SYMPTOMS

Tiredness and fatigue is commonly attributed to HIV infection and sometimes improve after the commencement of antiretroviral therapy. It may be the sole complaint of those with good immunity in whom antiretrovirals are not indicated. Investigation and treatment of conditions such as anaemia (common even in early disease) or co-existing medical conditions may be indicated if symptoms are severe or persistent. Consider mood disorder, hormonal deficiency (particularly sex hormones) and lifestyle factors including recreational drug use. Vitamin supplements may help and complementary therapies such as massage can improve general well-being. Night sweats may be particularly troublesome: regular paracetamol sometimes helps, but night sweats are notoriously difficult to control.

DERMATOLOGICAL PROBLEMS (Box 10.2)

The first clinical manifestation of HIV infection is often in the skin: typically seborrhoeic dermatitis. Prior to the use of HAART, 90% of HIV infected patients developed a dermatological condition and up to 40% had seborrhoeic dermatitis. An itchy, erythematous, scaly rash affecting the cheeks, nasolabial folds and forehead (Fig. 10.2), it may extend to other areas of the body especially at lower CD4 counts. The condition is very common in HIV-negative as well as HIV-positive individuals: the cause is probably the fungus *Malessezia furfur*, which can be isolated from skin scrapings if the diagnosis is uncertain. Psoriasis may appear for the first time after HIV acquisition, or become more problematic if it predates the infection. It may worsen (but sometimes remits) as immunosuppression progresses. Treatment is as in the non-HIV-infected individual. Staphylococcal and other bacterial skin infections including folliculitis, impetigo and recurrent abscesses can be problematic. Fungal infections including recurrent vaginal

Box 10.2: Dermatological infections in HIV

Condition	Principles of management	Example therapies
Seborrhoeic dermatitis	Use moisturisers, soap substitutes, topical azoles and steroids. Oral azole plus topical steroid (short course 2–4 weeks) if severe. May resolve (after an initial worsening) with HAART	Emollient cream. Mild: Canesten HC, Daktacort. Moderate: Betnovate C. Severe: Itraconazole 100 mg once daily plus Betnovate cream twice daily
Genital warts	As in HIV uninfected (Ch. 7). Aggressive treatment may be required	Cryotherapy. Topical podophyllotoxin. Topical imiquimod cream. Surgery
Molluscum contagiosum	Bacterial superinfection occurs – oral antibiotics. May improve with immune reconstitution	Cryotherapy. Topical podophyllotoxin
Herpes simplex	As HIV uninfected (Ch. 6) but for intermittent therapy use higher doses for longer duration (10 days). Higher doses may be required for suppressive therapy: Dose can be titrated to achieve suppression. Aciclovir resistance may occur	Intermittent therapy: Valaciclovir 1 g twice daily for 10 days. Suppressive therapy: Aciclovir 400–800 mg two to three times daily
Herpes zoster	As for HIV uninfected, but may be given for longer duration	Aciclovir 800 mg five times daily for 10 days

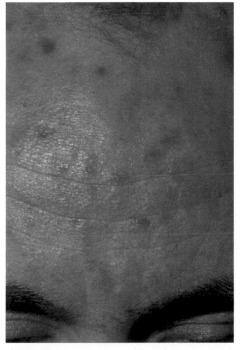

Figure 10.2
Seborrhoeic dermatitis of the forehead

candidiasis or intertrigo or tinea infection of the feet (Fig. 10.3), groin or nails are common. Viral infections are common early signs of deteriorating cellular immunity in the skin. Viral warts including genital (Fig. 10.4), plane and plantar warts may progress rapidly and to a large size. Molluscum contagiosum (Fig. 10.5) can also become extensive and secondarily infected. Herpes virus infections of the mouth and genitals are more frequent and more severe in HIV infection (Fig. 10.6). Herpetic ulcers may become chronic and persistent with advanced immunosuppression, constituting an AIDS diagnosis if they persist for more than a month. They are important not only because they are painful and debilitating, but because they potentially increase the risk of onward transmission of HIV to serodiscordant partners and acquisition of superinfection from other HIV-positive partners. The threshold for initiating suppressive therapy for HSV in people with HIV should be low. Herpes zoster (shingles) is a common manifestation of HIV disease, occurring at any stage. It may be atypical, affecting multiple dermatomes or presenting as disseminated infection (Fig. 10.7). As in the HIV uninfected, trigeminal zoster is an ophthalmic emergency: always consider the possibility in those with unusual

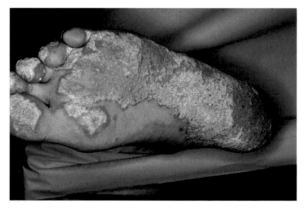

Figure 10.3
Tinea pedis in a man with HIV infection

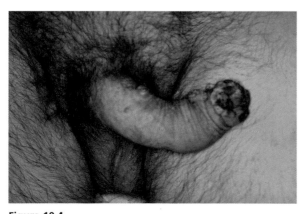

Figure 10.4
Massive genital warts in advanced immunosuppression

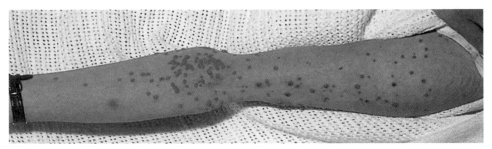

Figure 10.5
Secondarily infected molluscum contagiosum in HIV

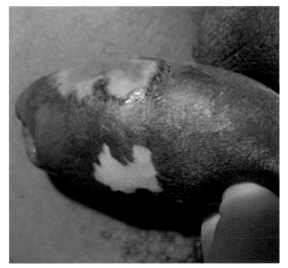

Figure 10.6
Frequently recurrent genital herpes with depigmentation

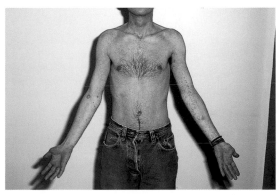

Figure 10.7
Bilateral multidermatomal zoster in untreated HIV infection

unilateral ocular or facial symptoms. Standard therapies are used for herpes virus infections in HIV, but higher doses are usually given for an extended duration.

ORAL LESIONS

Oral manifestations are common in early disease as well as with advanced immunosuppression (Box 10.3). Encourage dental review or make a dental referral soon after diagnosis as many patients have troublesome periodontal disease or gingivitis. Rarely this may progress to necrotizing ulcerative periodontitis, in which gingiva and bone is destroyed and teeth may be lost. Oral hairy leukoplakia (Fig. 10.8) presents as thickened, corrugated white plaque on the lateral margin of the tongue and is typical (though not pathognomonic) of HIV infection. It is caused by infection with EBV and is usually asymptomatic, requiring no treatment. Symptomatic white oral plaques are commonly due to the pseudomembranous form of oral candidiasis (Fig. 10.9). *Candida* infection may also present with angular cheilitis (cracking and splitting at the angles of the mouth) or with smooth erythematous patches or ulcers of the oral mucosa. Idiopathic recurrent aphthous ulcers are common: herpes virus infection, syphilis, thrush and rarely Kaposi's sarcoma or tonsillar lymphoma should always be considered in the differential diagnosis. Biopsy may be necessary if the diagnosis is in doubt.

Box 10.3: Oral manifestations of HIV infection

Condition	Notes on management	Example therapies
Gingivitis	Refer to dental surgeon, give antibiotics in the interim if painful and bleeding Severe disease (necrotizing ulcerative gingivitis) requires immediate attention	Metronidazole 400 mg three times daily for 5–7 days
Oral hairy leukoplakia	If asymptomatic no treatment May be a marker of rapid disease progression	Antivirals such as ganciclovir have been used
Oral candidiasis (thrush)	Treat episodically Resistance to fluconazole may occur (itraconazole is an alternative) Prophylactic therapy is not usually indicated but patients can be supplied with therapy to self-initiate in case of recurrence	Mild: Nystatin or amphotericin lozenges Moderate: fluconazole 150 mg once Severe: Fluconazole 50–100 mg once daily, ketoconazole 200 mg once daily or itraconazole 200 mg once daily for 7–14 days[1]
Recurrent oral herpes	As for genital herpes	See Box 6.12
Aphthous ulceration	Exclude other diagnoses Biopsy if diagnosis uncertain	Mild: Topical steroid e.g. Adcortyl in orabase Severe: thalidomide 100–200 mg once daily

[1]Ketoconazole is least expensive, but is affected by hepatic enzyme inducers and inhibitors (including some antiretrovirals) and is most hepatotoxic. Fluconazole is reliably absorbed and less hepatotoxic

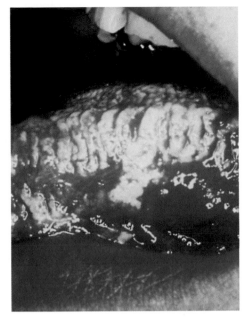

Figure 10.8
Oral hairy leukoplakia in advanced HIV infection

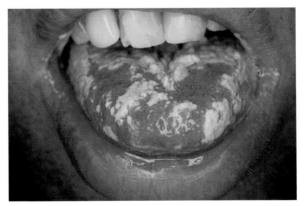

Figure 10.9
Oral candidiasis

PREVENTION OF OPPORTUNISTIC INFECTION

Prophylaxis against OI remains an important part of patient management and the only disease-modifying intervention available in many parts of the world. Prevention of the development of disease due to opportunistic infection may take the form of:

- behaviour change to avoid exposure to pathogens (e.g. *Toxoplasma*, *Cryptosporidium*)
- active immunization (e.g. against hepatitis B)

235

- passive immunization (e.g. against varicella zoster virus)
- a course of treatment for suspected latent infection (e.g. *Mycobacterium tuberculosis*)
- long-term chemoprophylaxis against the acquisition of pathogens in the community, or the development of disease due to pathogens previously acquired and carried without symptoms (e.g. PCP, CMV).

Primary prophylaxis against opportunistic infection is intervention to prevent a first episode of disease in someone at increased risk because of immunosuppression. It does not necessarily prevent acquisition of infection. Secondary prophylaxis is given to prevent recurrence following a first episode of illness. Prior to the advent of HAART, prophylaxis was usually continued for life. There is now evidence from randomized controlled trials that for PCP, *Toxoplasma* encephalitis and *Mycobacterium avium* complex (MAC), primary prophylaxis may be safely discontinued if sufficient immune recovery occurs with antiretroviral therapy. Recommendations for the discontinuation of primary prophylaxis for other infections (e.g. *Cryptococcus neoformans*, CMV) and for the discontinuation of secondary prophylaxis are based on cohort studies or expert opinion and remain subject to debate.

Initiation of chemoprophylaxis should be considered in all patients who have CD4 count measurements below the guideline thresholds for initiation. Exceptions are sometimes made, for example when HAART is initiated at just below the threshold for prophylaxis. The most comprehensive guidelines are those of the US Public Health Service (USPHS) and Infectious Diseases Society of America. Box 10.4 and Box 10.5 contain brief summaries of main recommendations.

AIDS

The probability of major opportunistic infection or other AIDS-defining condition increases with deterioration in immune function. The initial outpatient assessment of common symptoms and diagnosis of the most frequently encountered conditions is described here. As discussed in Chapter 10, the majority of new AIDS diagnoses in the UK are made simultaneous with or soon after an HIV diagnosis, so the assessment of symptoms may well be made on first presentation, before a CD4 count is available or sometimes without a positive HIV antibody result.

RESPIRATORY DISEASE

Pneumocystis carinii pneumonia (commonly referred to as PCP although the organism has been renamed *Pneumocystis jiroveci*) is the commonest respiratory condition in AIDS (Fig. 10.10). It is usually seen at CD4 count below 200 cells/mm^3 in people not taking

Box 10.4: Prevention of opportunistic infection

Organism	Prevention
Pneumocystis carinii	Ubiquitous organism: no evidence exposure can be avoided Primary and secondary chemoprophylaxis
Mycobacterium tuberculosis	Avoid high-risk occupations (e.g. with the homeless) – little evidence Tuberculin skin test at diagnosis if at risk. If positive and no evidence of active TB, treatment for latent TB
Toxoplasma gondii	If toxoplasma IgG negative at diagnosis, avoid raw or undercooked red meat. Infectious form takes several days to develop after excretion so change cat-litter daily. Wash hands after gardening, wash fruit and vegetables. Retest seronegative individuals if CD4 <100. Primary and secondary chemoprophylaxis
Mycobacterium avium complex	Ubiquitous organism: no evidence exposure can be avoided Primary and secondary chemoprophylaxis
Varicella zoster virus	Avoid exposure to chickenpox or shingles Confirm a history of chickenpox or shingles at diagnosis, do VZV IgG serology if no history VZV immunoglobulin if exposed and seronegative
Bacterial respiratory infections: *Streptococcus pneumoniae* *Haemophilus influenzae*	Exposure cannot be avoided Polyvalent pneumococcal vaccine is recommended for all HIV infected people (although this is contrary to the available evidence). *Haemophilus influenza* type B (HiB) vaccine not recommended
Cryptosporidium spp.	Boil drinking water for 1 minute during outbreaks Some recommend boiling or filtering all drinking water at all times as a precaution
Hepatitis A Hepatitis B Influenza virus	Vaccinate at diagnosis or defer until CD4 count improves if HAART initiated (Ch. 9)
Cryptococcus neoformans *Histoplasma capsulatum* Cytomegalovirus	Secondary chemoprophylaxis recommended Primary chemoprophylaxis not routinely recommended

HAART, but should be considered at higher CD4 counts in patients with typical symptoms or where no other diagnosis is found. The onset is insidious and clinical chest signs are uncommon – a low threshold for investigation is appropriate in those at risk (Box 10.6). PCP should also be considered in those taking PCP prophylaxis – the presentation in these cases may be acute and X-ray findings atypical. Bacterial pneumonia in people with HIV infection is increased in incidence between 6- and 20-fold (Fig. 10.11) compared to the non-HIV-infected population, so should always be included in the differential diagnosis of respiratory symptoms. The incidence of bacterial pneumonia is also related to the CD4 count and around 50% is due to *S. pneumoniae*. Although pulmonary tuberculosis may present at any CD4 count, typical symptoms and signs are

Box 10.5: Primary prophylaxis against opportunistic infection

Condition	First-line prophylactic regimen[1]	Initiate at	Discontinue at
Pneumocystis carinii	Cotrimoxazole 480–960 mg once daily or Cotrimoxazole 960 mg three times a week	CD4 <200 cells/mm^3 or 14%, or oropharyngeal candidiasis	CD4 >200 cells/mm^3 for 3 months
Toxoplasma gondii	Oral regimens for PCP are active against *Toxoplasma*	If *Toxoplasma* IgG seropositive at CD4 <100 cells/mm^3	CD4 >200 cells/mm^3 for 3 months
Mycobacterium tuberculosis	Isoniazid 300 mg once daily plus pyridoxine 50 mg once daily	Positive TST or exposure to MTB with no evidence of active disease	Treat for 9 months
Mycobacterium avium complex	Azithromycin 1250 mg once weekly OR clarithromycin 500 mg orally twice daily	CD4 <50cells/mm^3	CD4 >100cells/mm^3 for 3 months
Varicella zoster virus (VZV)	Varicella zoster immune globulin (VZIG) five vials of 1.25 ml	Confirmed exposure to VZV and no history of chickenpox/shingles, VZV IgG negative	Single-dose treatment

[1]First-line regimen only included. There are multiple satisfactory alternatives.

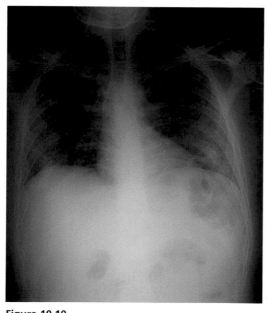

Figure 10.10
Pneumocystis carinii pneumonia

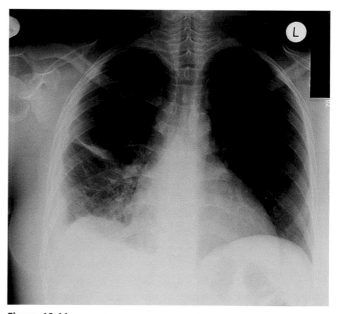

Figure 10.11
Reactive pleural effusion due to bacterial pneumonia in HIV

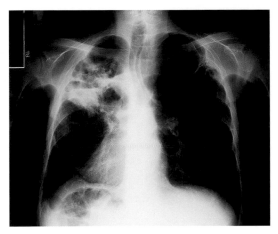

Figure 10.12
Cavitating lesion of tuberculosis in HIV

more likely to be seen when the immune system is relatively intact (CD4 >300 cells/mm^3): atypical features and disseminated disease are more likely with increasing immunosuppression (Fig. 10.12). The implications of untreated pulmonary TB for the patient and their HIV-positive and negative contacts make the early diagnosis or exclusion of TB of the highest priority (Box 10.7). Less common conditions that may be included in the differential diagnosis of the HIV-positive patient with respiratory symptoms are tracheal or bronchial candidiasis, pulmonary Kaposi's sarcoma (very rare without cutaneous lesions) and lymphoma. Pulmonary cryptococcosis, aspergillosis and MAI occur in advanced disease (usually when the CD4 count is <50 cells/mm^3). Upper respiratory infections and particularly sinusitis are common at all stages of HIV infection.

Clinical features

History

Onset of symptoms: a gradual onset with reduced exercise tolerance, dry cough and breathlessness over several weeks suggests PCP. An acute onset is more typical of a community-acquired bacterial pneumonia.

Cough: a non- or minimally-productive cough suggests PCP, purulent sputum a bacterial cause. Bloodstaining or frank haemoptysis may be a symptom of TB, fungal infection or malignancy

Accompanying symptoms: systemic symptoms including weight loss may be seen with both PCP and tuberculosis. Pleuritic chest pain and night sweats are typical of pulmonary TB.

Examination

Chest signs are rarely helpful in the diagnosis of PCP, except that their absence in the patient with severe symptoms may indicate the diagnosis. Occasionally fine 'cellophane' crackles may be heard, but more usually there are no signs. PCP occasionally presents with a pneumothorax. It is rarely diagnosed in patients without other signs of immunosuppression: oral candidiasis or seborrhoeic dermatitis are likely.

Signs of lobar consolidation, collapse or pleural effusion may be seen with bacterial pneumonia but always consider the possibility of TB. A pleural effusion may be reactive or due to TB, Kaposi's sarcoma or lymphoma.

Investigation

Investigation is as in the HIV-negative patient, but be alert to atypical presentations of common pathogens and the possibility of dual pathology. Consider common bacterial respiratory pathogens and opportunistic infections according to CD4 count. Figure 10.13 outlines the outpatient assessment of a patient with respiratory symptoms.

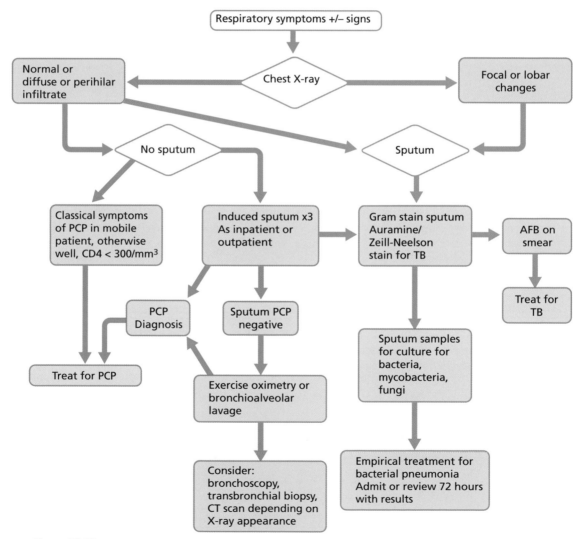

Figure 10.13
Outpatient assessment of respiratory symptoms

- Full blood count
- Chest X-ray
- Blood cultures if pyrexial
- Sputum for staining for microscopy for bacteria, MTB and fungi (request Indian ink stain for cryptococcus if CD4 <50)
- Sputum culture and sensitivity for bacteria, mycobacteria, fungi
- Atypical titres (*Legionella pneumophila, Chlamydia psittaci, Mycoplasma pneumoniae, Coxiella burnetti*)
- Pulse oximetry

Consider
- Arterial blood gas analysis
- Pneumococcal antigen (countercurrent immunoelectrophoresis)
- Sputum cytology
- Lactate dehydrogenase
- Exercise pulse oximetry
- Induced sputum for staining, immunofluorescence or PCR for PCP and/or staining for MTB ($\times$ 3 sequential samples, can sometimes be performed as an outpatient)
- Broncheoalveolar lavage

Management

Standard markers for the assessment of pneumonia (respiratory rate, blood pressure, oxygen saturation) plus consideration of the CD4 count and X-ray findings will indicate whether outpatient management can be considered, or immediate hospital admission for further investigation and treatment is required. The initial management of PCP is outlined in Box 10.6 and of TB in Box 10.7.

Case history

Blessing is a 33-year-old Zambian man who reluctantly attends a walk-in clinic at an HIV centre. He has previously taken antiretroviral therapy for his HIV infection. He was lost to follow-up and discontinued therapy 2 years previously when his CD4 count was 265 cells/mm^3. He has a non-productive cough and has become breathless on exercise over the last 6 weeks. He has no clinical signs on chest examination, but has oral candidiasis. There is minimal increase in interstitial markings on chest X-ray. He has an oxygen saturation of 93% on air, but desaturates to 85% on exercise. He absolutely refuses to be admitted to hospital as he fears that this will expose his HIV status to his family. A presumptive diagnosis of PCP is made. He is commenced on 3 weeks of co-trimoxazole 960 mg, two tablets, four times daily, plus fluconazole 100 mg once daily. He is warned of possible side effects and encouraged to re-attend promptly if he fails to improve.

NEUROLOGICAL DISEASE

As with other bacterial infections, bacterial meningitis and pyogenic abscess are seen with increased frequency in those with HIV and may occur at any CD4 count. Neurological complications of opportunistic infections and malignancy are uncommon at CD4 count over 200 cells/mm^3 and the differential diagnosis of the patient presenting with CNS symptoms can be modified according to the CD4 count. The OI most commonly affecting the CNS is *Toxoplasma gondii* infection (Fig. 10.14). Its symptoms; those of a focal brain lesion with mass effect and radiological findings of ring-enhancing lesions on CT scan are often indistinguishable from the important differential diagnosis: primary intracerebral

Box 10.6: Pneumocystis carinii

Disease	Pneumonia (common)
	Retinitis (uncommon)
Diagnosis/investigation	Pneumonia: Presumptive on clinical findings, CXR and pulse oximetry or by induced sputum: inhaled 3% saline and deep coughing
	Exercise oximetry: 3% fall from baseline after 10 minutes
	Bronchoalveolar lavage (BAL)
Identification	*Pneumocystis jiroveci* in induced sputum specimens by staining, immunofluorescence or PCR
Treatment (first-line)	Co-trimoxazole (trimethoprim and sulphamethoxazole) 120 mg/kg/day in divided doses either orally or i.v. for 21 days
	Two 960 mg tablets of co-trimoxazole four times daily is the typical dose for outpatient treatment
	Rash and nausea are very common side effects; Treatment may be continued if symptoms are relieved by antihistamines and antiemetics
	Monitor for neutropaenia and thrombocytopaenia
	Give corticosteroids if PaO2 on air <9.3kPa or 70 mmHg. Prednisolone 40 mg twice daily for 5 days, 20 mg twice daily for 5 days, 20 mg once daily for 11 days

Box 10.7: Mycobacterium tuberculosis

Disease	Localized pulmonary disease (upper lobe) if CD4 >300
	Disseminated pulmonary disease, brain, visceral involvement with advancing immunosuppression
Investigation/diagnosis	Smears of expectorated/induced sputum on 3 consecutive days (detects 90% of pulmonary TB)
	Presumptive diagnosis: AFB on Auramine or Ziehl-Neelsen stains of sputum
Identification	Culture or molecular techniques (applied to pleural, lymph node, bone marrow, transbronchial or other biopsy specimens)
	Standard culture media (8 weeks to identification) or rapid systems (e.g. BACTEC – 2 weeks)
	Molecular diagnostic techniques such as PCR. PCR is less sensitive on non-pulmonary specimens
Treatment (first-line)	Always in conjunction with microbiologist and a physician with experience of TB management
	Directly observed therapy preferred – mandatory if MDR-TB
	Rifampicin, isonazid, pyrazinamide and ethambutol for 2 months, then rifampicin and isoniazid continued for 6 months (12 months in miliary or meningeal disease)
	Up to six drugs may be used in suspected multi-drug resistant MDR-TB): Mortality is very high in MDR-TB

lymphoma (Fig. 10.15). Mass lesions due to systemic lymphoma or other systemic infections (cryptococcus, tuberculosis, staphylococcus) are more usually seen as complications than as the initial manifestation of these diagnoses. Progressive multifocal leukoencephalopathy (PML) is a disease of white matter caused by infection with the JC virus, usually with advanced immunosuppression, in which focal lesions occur without mass effect; presentation may also be with focal neurological signs but headache is uncommon. Cytomegalovirus (CMV) infection of the CNS (Fig. 10.16) most commonly

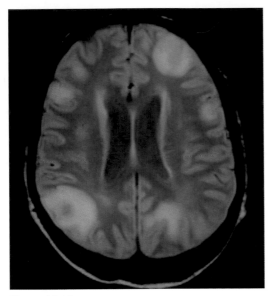

Figure 10.14
MRI showing multiple lesions of cerebral toxoplasmosis

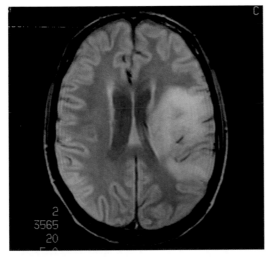

Figure 10.15
MRI of primary CNS lymphoma

presents with visual field loss or 'floaters' due to CMV retinitis in those with CD4 <100 cells/mm^3 (Box 10.9). CMV encephalitis is rare. The pathogenic effects of HIV itself, without the involvement of opportunistic organisms, are seen in the nervous system. AIDS dementia complex is a common late manifestation of HIV, occurring in around 20% of those with AIDS prior to the use of HAART (Fig. 10.17). Initially, very soft signs of changes in behaviour or mild cognitive and motor impairment are rapidly progressive to eventual dementia and quadriplegia without treatment.

243

Peripheral sensory neuropathy due to HIV infection is common in advanced disease. Antiretroviral drugs (especially didanosine) and vinca alkaloids used for the treatment of lymphoma or Kaposi's sarcoma may exacerbate the condition.

Clinical features

Many patients present with mild symptoms of gradual onset and early recognition of intracerebral pathology affects outcomes. Classic symptoms and signs of CNS infection such as meningism may be atypical or absent. Patients with moderate or severe immunosuppression who present with seizure, new onset headache, visual changes or focal neurological signs should be immediately and fully assessed. If in doubt about the significance of CNS symptoms in the immunosuppressed patient with absent or minimal clinical signs, it is usually wise to arrange a CT (or MRI) brain scan (see Fig. 10.18).

History

Focal infective or malignant lesions may present with seizures, rapid onset of confusion or changes in motor power, sensation or co-ordination. Frontal headache with or without

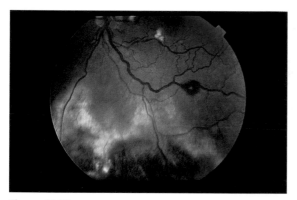

Figure 10.16
CMV retinitis

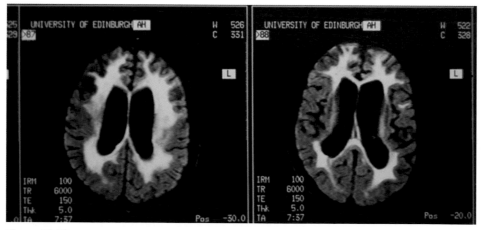

Figure 10.17
Progression of cortical atrophy with HIV dementia

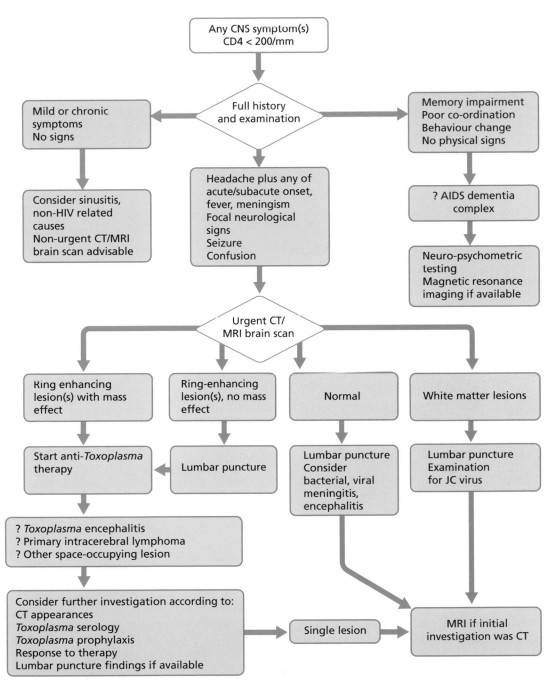

Figure 10.18
Initial assessment of neurological symptoms

facial pain may be due to sinusitis – very common in HIV infection at all CD4 counts. Loss of part of the visual field or 'floaters' in a patient with CD4 <100 cells/mm^3 should raise the possibility of cytomegalovirus retinitis (Box 10.9). Although loss of concentration and memory impairment are early signs of HIV dementia, they are also common features of mood disorder. Conversely, changes in mood and behaviour may also be early signs of dementia, which should always be considered if such symptoms present at low CD4 count. Well-informed patients at low risk of dementia may be anxious regarding such symptoms and appropriate investigation can provide reassurance.

Examination

Although physical examination is rarely diagnostic, if thorough and accurately documented at presentation it may be very useful in assessing the response (or lack of response) to empirical treatment. This may be particularly important in deciding on further investigation or changes in therapy.

Investigation

Baseline investigation of the patient with headache, seizure or focal neurological symptoms or signs should include:

- full blood count
- blood cultures and throat swab (if pyrexial)
- syphilis serology
- CT or MRI scan according to availability
- lumbar puncture if not contra-indicated by scan findings
- *Toxoplasma* serology, if the CD4 count is <200 cells/mm^3, and serum cryptococcal antigen, if the CD4 count is <100 cells/mm^3.

Consider:

- mycobacterial cultures (blood, stool, urine)
- CT with sinus views
- dental review.

Management

The management of *Toxoplasma* encephalitis is outlined in Box 10.8. Cranial irradiation and steroid therapy is given in primary CNS lymphoma but the prognosis remains poor. The progression of PML and AIDS dementia is retarded and has been reported to reverse with antiretroviral therapy.

GASTROINTESTINAL DISEASE

Common presentations of gastrointestinal disease in HIV include dysphagia, wasting and diarrhoea. Acute diarrhoea due to enteric infection (usually food poisoning) with *Salmonella*, *Shigella* and *Campylobacter* may be seen at any stage of HIV, as may

Clinical notes: lumbar puncture in HIV

Send samples for:
- Microscopy:
  Gram stain (cell count, bacteria)
  Auramine/ZN for mycobacteria
- Culture:
  Bacteria
  Mycobacteria
- Syphilis serology
- Biochemistry (protein)
- Glucose (with plasma glucose)
- Cytology

If CD4 <200:
- Indian-ink for *Cryptococcus*
- CSF cryptococccal antigen
- *Toxoplasma* antibody titre
- Herpes virus PCR

Consider:
- PCR for JC virus
- PCR for CMV
- PCR for Epstein–Barr virus (EBV)

Box 10.8: Toxoplasma gondii

Disease	Encephalitis with focal mass lesions Pneumonitis, retinitis
Investigation/diagnosis	Ring enhancing lesion(s) on CT or MRI scan: initiate trial of anti-toxo therapy Lumbar puncture rarely possible. Diagnosis confirmed if symptoms and CT changes resolve on therapy: usually 2–3 weeks to improvement, 1–6 months to resolution
Identification	Positive *Toxoplasma* IgG supports diagnosis, negative does not exclude it PCR on CSF, PET scanning or stereotactic brain biopsy may be indicated if no improvement with empirical therapy
Treatment (first-line)	Sulphadiazine 2 g orally/i.v. 4 times a day Pyrimethamine 75 mg/day Folinic acid 15 mg/day Skin rash and neutropenia common

---

Clostridium difficile infection, particularly following antibiotic therapy. *Giardia intestinalis* presents with subacute symptoms and is common in men who have sex with men (MSM). Infection with the protozoans *Cryptosporidium* or *Microsporidia* causes chronic diarrhoea in patients with advanced immunosuppression (usually CD4 count of <200 cells/mm^3 and not taking HAART). The malabsorption and small-bowel dysfunction accompanying these infections contributes to the appearance of starvation in advanced untreated AIDS. *Cryptosporidium* cannot be eradicated by available antibacterials, but is eradicated by the recovery in immunity with successful antiretroviral therapy. The differential diagnosis of chronic diarrhoea expands with declining CD4 count and includes *Mycobacterium avium intracellulare* and cytomegalovirus, although in about one-third of cases, no cause is found. Oesophageal candidiasis is the commonest opportunistic infection affecting the GI tract and patients who have odynophagia, dysphagia or retrosternal discomfort should be treated empirically with antifungals. Ulceration due to cytomegalovirus, herpes simplex virus infection or drug side effects may present with similar symptoms, as may Kaposi's sarcoma, so patients who do not respond quickly and completely to antifungal therapy should undergo endoscopy.

Clinical features

Gastrointestinal side effects of antiretroviral and other drugs are particularly common and iatrogenic causes should always be considered in the differential diagnosis. For example, diarrhoea is particularly common with nelfinavir, ritonavir and didanosine, but infectious causes of diarrhoea may affect patients taking antiretroviral therapy who have persisting impaired immunity. Weight loss usually only occurs with advanced HIV or opportunistic infection. Patients complaining of weight loss on HAART may prove to be describing features of early lipoatrophy (Ch. 11). Recording accurate weights at baseline and at each clinic visit helps in determining the appropriate investigations in such cases – if weight loss is confirmed, investigation for opportunistic infection should be considered. Wasting may be assessed by simple anthropometry although Dexa scanning and 3-D imaging techniques are increasingly available, driven largely by interest in the assessment of lipodystrophy.

History

Painful swallowing or dysphagia are classical symptoms of oesophageal candidiasis, although a retrosternal discomfort or anorexia and the loss of taste sensation due to accompanying oral candidiasis may be the only clues to the diagnosis. Review changes to HIV and non-HIV medication in all cases. In those presenting with diarrhoea, assess the frequency (at least 3 × per day) of loose stool. A dietary, travel and drug history are vital in acute and chronic diarrhoea, and a history of oro–anal sex may be relevant in MSM (*Giardia intestinalis*, *Shigella* and others).

Examination

Oesophageal candidiasis is usually but not invariably associated with oral plaques. Examination is otherwise as in the HIV-uninfected patient.

Investigation

A trial of antifungal therapy (as for severe oral candidiasis – Box 10.3) is usually worthwhile before arranging an endoscopy in patients with suspected oesophageal *Candida*.

Stool analysis for ova, cysts and parasites including special stains for *Cryptosporidium* and *Microsporidia* is sufficient for the diagnosis of diarrhoea in patients with CD4 count of >200 cells/mm^3. It may need to be repeated 3–6 times to isolate *Cryptosporidium*. Rectal biopsy for diagnosis of cytomegalovirus and mycobacterial infection should be

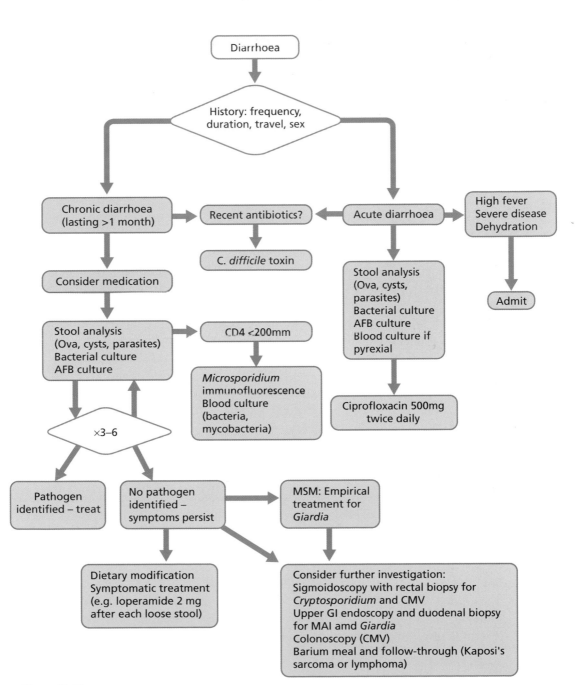

Figure 10.19
Outpatient assessment of neurological symptoms

considered if CD4 count is less than 100 cells/mm^3. Further investigations are outlined in Figure 10.19.

LIVER DISEASE

Hepatitis B and C share routes of transmission with HIV. Between 2% and 9% of all HIV infected patients are HBsAg positive. Some antiretroviral drugs are also active against hepatitis B (lamivudine, tenofovir) and the choice of HAART regimen in patients with HIV and chronic hepatitis B should be made with both infections in mind. Approximately 4–8% of homosexual men and 60–80% of IVDUs with HIV are co-infected with hepatitis C. As death rates from opportunistic infections reduce, an increasing proportion of deaths in HIV are due to liver failure in hepatitis co-infected patients. Recent reports suggest that 30–50% of deaths in HAART-treated cohorts are due to hepatitis C and many of these deaths occur in patients with well-controlled HIV infection. HIV appears to increase the HCV viral load, the rate of progression and the risk of cirrhosis and hepatocellular carcinoma. It is not clear at present whether hepatitis C infection also accelerates the course of HIV disease. The success rate of treatment with interferon monotherapy in co-infected patients was poor, but results with combination therapy with pegylated interferon and ribavirin appear comparable to those in non-HIV-infected patients, the initial response rate approaching 50% in HCV genotype 1 infection and up to 80% in genotypes 2 and 3. Interactions between antiretrovirals and hepatitis therapy mean that combination therapy may be difficult, but this does not preclude treatment. Horizontal and vertical transmission of hepatitis C transmission is increased 3–5-fold with HIV.

HIV-RELATED MALIGNANCY

The incidence of Kaposi's sarcoma and non-Hodgkins lymphoma are increased 100-fold in people with AIDS. The incidence of other malignancies including skin cancers, cervical and anal carcinoma, and lung adenocarcinoma is also increased. The decline in incidence of opportunistic infections observed following the introduction of HAART was also seen in Kaposi's sarcoma, but not initially in NHL. There is now some evidence of a delayed and less dramatic fall in cases of NHL. In clinical practice, the reduction in infectious complications of AIDS means that NHL has been observed to be responsible for a similar number, but a much greater proportion of patients presenting with symptoms (for example respiratory symptoms) than was previously the case.

Kaposi's sarcoma

AIDS-associated Kaposi's sarcoma (KS) is the most common AIDS-associated cancer (Fig. 10.20). It may occur at any CD4 count, although it is more frequently encountered with increasing immunosuppression. An essential cofactor in oncogenesis is human herpes virus 8 (HHV8), found in all KS lesions. HHV8 infection and KS is more common in MSM and African populations than in heterosexual caucasian HIV-infected patients. KS may present as pink, brown or purplish firm nodules, or less commonly plaques, anywhere on the skin surface, on the palate, or on epithelial surfaces in the gut, lung or

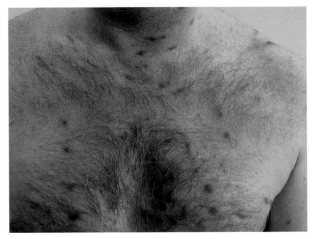

Figure 10.20
Kaposi's sarcoma

Box 10.9: Cytomegalovirus

Disease	Systemic infection at CD4 less than 50 cells/mm^3. Asymptomatic or manifests as retinitis, oesophageal ulceration, diarrhoea due to colitis, adrenalitis
Investigation/diagnosis	Retinitis: clinical diagnosis by ophthalmologist GI manifestations: biopsy Encephalitis: clinical diagnosis +/- CMV DNA in CSF
Identification	CMV IgG (nearly always positive) confirms previous exposure Histological examination of biopsy specimens for 'owl eye' inclusions PCR for CMV DNA in blood, CSF or biopsy specimens High titres of CMV DNA on quantitative PCR may indicate need for treatment in asymptomatic patients
Treatment (first-line)	Ganciclovir i.v. 10 mg/kg/day in induction, 5 mg/kg/day maintenance Ganciclovir 3 g/day orally as maintenance

body cavities. Treatment for solitary lesions may be with intralesional chemotherapy or local radiotherapy, but systemic chemotherapy with liposomal daunorubicin or doxorubicin is given for extensive or visceral disease. Paclitaxel is sometimes effective where first-line therapy fails.

Non-Hodgkin's lymphoma (NHL)

Diffuse large-cell lymphoma and small-cell Burkitt's lymphoma are seen in association with HIV infection. About half are associated with Epstein–Barr virus (EBV), although primary intracerebral lymphoma is invariably associated with EBV. HIV associated NHL is often extranodal and commonly presents with advanced disease. B symptoms such as night sweats, fatigue and weight loss are usual, and it is important to be alert to the possibility of lymphoma in patients who develop new non-specific systemic symptoms when otherwise stable on antiretroviral therapy. Other presentations include painful lymphadenopathy or pain or symptoms of obstruction of the respiratory or gastrointestinal tract, due to local node involvement. CT scan of the thorax, abdomen and pelvis, plus lymph node biopsy and bone marrow examination are needed for diagnosis and staging. The previously dire prognosis has improved significantly with the combination of HAART and chemotherapy.

PALLIATIVE CARE

The number of AIDS cases and deaths have reduced dramatically in developed nations since 1995, but late diagnosis is common and HIV remains an incurable infection. Palliative care in HIV medicine cannot be regarded as end-of-life care. Many patients may have long periods of severe illness, sometimes immediately after diagnosis, which may be followed by death or by full recovery. Palliative care in AIDS often involves highly active intervention as well as symptom control. See Further reading for guidance on pain control and symptom management.

Clinical notes: palliative care

- Advance directives or living wills should be part of routine care.
- The involvement of palliative care specialists should be considered early – not at the point of withdrawing active treatment.
- Quality of life is important and subjective, but measurable using standard scales. It may change dramatically with increasing disability.
- Pain is underdiagnosed and treated, particularly in mobile patients.
- Fatigue and lack of sleep are commonly overlooked symptoms in HIV infection.
- Social factors (homelessness, money, care of partner or children) may be additional stressors.
- Patients from outside the UK may have additional cultural and language barriers to care and lack family and community support.
- The stigma attached to HIV/AIDS persists and may affect the patient's attitude to place of care (e.g. AIDS hospice or ward) and disclosure to relatives.

Further Reading

Bruno R, Sacchi P, Puoti M, Soriano V, Filice G. HCV chronic hepatitis in patients with HIV: Clinical management issues. Am Jour Gastro 2002; 97: 1598–1606.

Fauci AS, Pantaleo G, Stanley S, Weismann D. Immunopathogenic mechanisms of HIV infection. Ann Intern Med 1996; 124: 654–63.

Gazzard B (ed). AIDS Care Handbook. London; Mediscript: 2002.

Havlir DV, Barnes PF. Tuberculosis in patients with human immunodeficiency virus infection. N Engl J Med 1999; 340: 367–373.

Meyer M. Palliative care and AIDS: 1 – Pain. Int Jour STD & AIDS 1999; 10: 80–88.

Meyer M. Palliative care and AIDS: 2 – Gastrointestinal symptoms. Int Jour STD & AIDS 1999; 10: 495–507.

Poles MA, Dietrich DT. Hepatitis C virus/ human immunodeficiency virus coinfection: Clinical management issues. Clin Inf Dis 2000; 31: 154–61.

Posniak A. The management of opportunistic infections in AIDS. In: Barton SE, Hay PE (eds). Handbook of genitourinary medicine. London; Arnold: 1999.

Tschachler E, Bergstresser PR, Stingl G. HIV-related skin diseases. Lancet 1996; 348: 659–653.

Wolff AJ, O'Donnell, AE. Pulmonary manifestations of HIV infection in the era of highly active antiretroviral therapy. Chest 2001; 120: 1888–1893.

SELF-ASSESSMENT

Clara is a 35-year-old South African woman who has been under care for her HIV infection for 7 years. She has taken multiple antiretroviral regimens and finds it difficult to take her medication regularly. At her last clinic visit, 4 weeks ago, she was well and received nebulized pentamidine as prophylaxis against PCP. Her CD4 count had fallen to 85 cells/mm^3 and her viral load was 28 000 copies/ml on therapy. Her 17-year-old son brings her to the HIV outpatient clinic. She has become acutely confused over the past 3 days. She is disorientated and agitated.

Questions
a) What investigations would you order and why?
b) An urgent CT scan shows two lesions in the right cerebral hemisphere with contrast enhancement and midline shift. Which two facts from her previous casenotes would be most useful?
c) What treatment would you give?

Answers
a) Baseline investigations include: full blood count, blood cultures (exclude sepsis), pulse oximetry, X-ray (hypoxia due to respiratory infection), urea and electrolytes (uraemia, liver failure, drug toxicity), glucose (hypoglycaemia), syphilis serology, cryptococcal antigen, mycobacterial cultures.
b) *Toxoplasma* serology result and whether anti-*Toxoplasma* prophylaxis is prescribed. She is *Toxoplasma* IgG positive and she has been receiving inhaled pentamidine at a dose of 300 mg once monthly as prophylaxis against *Pneumocystis carinii* pneumonia. This is not effective as prophylaxis against *Toxoplasma gondii*.
c) Start treatment for presumed *Toxoplasma* encephalitis. Most clinicians would do so even if she was *Toxoplasma* IgG negative and was receiving anti-*Toxoplasma* prophylaxis, although this would make the diagnosis much less likely. Sulphadiazine 100 mg/kg orally or intravenously four times daily plus pyrimethamine 75 mg orally once daily. Steroid therapy may reduce oedema and relieve symptoms but does not improve outcome.

Antiretroviral therapy

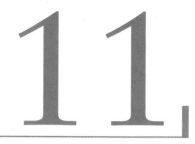

BACKGROUND

From the licensing of zidovudine for the treatment of HIV in 1987, the number of available drugs and the complexity of management have gradually increased. Concern about lack of access to antiretroviral therapy, both by socially marginalized groups in developed nations and by the vast majority of those affected by HIV in developing nations, has politicized people with HIV/AIDS to an extent previously unseen in any group affected by a single disease. Although the use of mono and then dual therapy was shown to improve clinical outcomes, it was in 1996 that the administration of three or more antiretroviral drugs simultaneously, as 'triple combination' or 'highly-active antiretroviral therapy' (HAART) was recognized to transform the natural history of AIDS. The antiretrovirals available in 2003 can be grouped by mechanism of action into five main classes and drugs from one or more groups may be used together. For a short time in the late 1990s there was hope that by using HAART, with or without adjunctive therapies, HIV could be eradicated from the individual. The incorporation of the HIV genome into the cellular DNA of long-lived cells of the immune system has so far proved an insurmountable obstacle to achieving this goal. At present, antiretroviral therapy is regarded as long-term, possibly lifelong treatment. The clinical benefit of antiretroviral therapy in those with symptomatic disease is proven beyond doubt. The timing of initiation of therapy in asymptomatic patients, the choice of drugs and the sequence in which they are used is more controversial. Recommendations for best practice continue to develop quite rapidly and there have been significant differences in approach between the USA and much of Europe.

The urgency with which treatment was required and the pressure appropriately applied by representatives of the affected community has meant that new therapies have been used therapeutically at relatively early stages of development. Both long-term and rarer short term adverse effects may only come to light after drugs have been in widespread use for some time. In HIV therapy these have included metabolic disturbances involving dyslipidaemia and insulin resistance, changes in body shape (lipodystrophy) and peripheral neuropathy. The management of debilitating long-term side effects has become an increasingly important component of HIV management where antiretrovirals are available. These tolerability factors, plus the difficulties involved in sustaining regular pill taking, and the dietary and other lifestyle restrictions involved in taking HAART, have made the issue of adherence to therapy a major concern in HIV management.

PATHOGENESIS AND CLINICAL PRACTICE

Antiretroviral drugs achieve their common end of inhibiting HIV replication by interrupting the HIV life-cycle at various stages (Fig. 11.1).

Nucleoside analogue reverse transcriptase-inhibitors ('nucleosides' or NRTIs) are modified versions of naturally occurring cellular nucleosides. These are purine and pyrimidine bases attached to pentagonal sugars that when further phosphorylated by intracellular enzymes become nucleotides: the unitary components of DNA and RNA. Nucleoside analogues such as azidothymidine (usually called zidovudine or AZT) are recognized as natural nucleosides by the viral enzyme reverse transcriptase and are incorporated into the evolving DNA chain. They lack a terminal hydroxy group essential for continuation of the nucleotide helix and are, therefore, chain-terminators.

Nucleotide drugs (e.g. tenofovir) act in a similar way to NRTIs but enter the cell in a phosphorylated form.

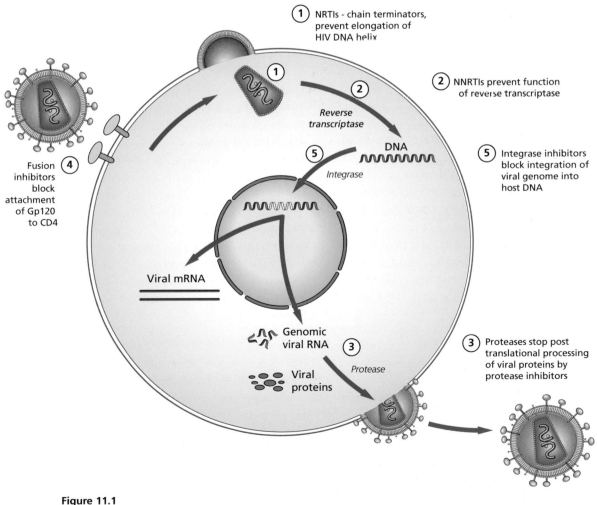

Figure 11.1
Sites of action of antiretroviral drugs

Non-nucleoside reverse transcriptase inhibitors (NNRTIs) (e.g. nevirapine) bind to the reverse transcriptase enzyme and cause a conformational change inhibiting function.

Protease inhibitors (PIs) (e.g. ritonavir) contain analogues of a vital section of HIV protein recognized by another enzyme, HIV protease.

Fusion inhibitors (e.g enfuvirtide (T20)) prevent binding of HIV to the CD4 cell surface.

Integrase inhibitors (none yet licensed) prevent the incorporation of the completed HIV DNA copy into the host cell DNA.

The interruption of the HIV replicative life cycle and the short lifespan of infective virions means that after starting antiretroviral therapy the viral load falls rapidly ($1\log_{10}$ every 10 days). With a reduction in viral load, there is reduced immune system activation reflected in lower levels of activation markers (such as TNF-α), less destruction of CD4 cells and reduced catabolism. In the treatment of AIDS this may be paralleled by improved well-being, recovery from infections, weight gain and better quality of life. If reduction in viral load is maintained, immune recovery can occur, with improvements at first in memory CD4 cells and later in some naïve CD4 cell populations. Immune reconstitution can also cause illness: longstanding infection may be unmasked when the regenerating immune system mounts a response causing symptoms.

HIV reverse transcriptase does not possess a 3-prime to 5-prime 'proofreading' ability. It is unable to correct the many genetic 'mistakes', or substitutions of one nucleotide for another, made in the process of producing new copies of the viral genome. These mistakes are translated into amino-acid substitutions in viral proteins and, hence, structural or functional changes in the virus. Each individual carries a number of populations of HIV or quasispecies – each genetically different. In the natural state, the predominant quasispecies is 'wild-type' virus: virus with the genotype encoding the most effective phenotype for the environment. Genotypic mutations affecting replicative capacity, cell attachment or viral processing place a viral quasispecies at a selective disadvantage and the population of such viruses remains small. However, certain genetic mistakes, or mutations, will, by chance, affect antiretroviral processing, transport, binding or function. Viruses with such mutations will have a survival advantage in the presence of such drugs and become the predominant viral species.

The high frequency with which mutations occur results in every possible mutation (and double mutation) being produced in an infected individual every day. Some of these mutations confer drug resistance. In the presence of one or two drugs, a drug-resistant viral strain rapidly becomes dominant and the antiretroviral effect is short-lived. However, the chance of sufficient mutations occurring to confer resistance to three drugs administered simultaneously is low. Three or more drugs may suppress viral replication sufficiently (and in some cases completely) and thus prevent the emergence of resistance for as long as the drugs are taken.

Mutations that allow the virus to resist drug effects also have some disadvantageous effect for the virus (otherwise viruses with the mutation would have become the predominant strain by natural selection). A drug resistant virus may, therefore, be 'unfit' – less able to replicate, or less able to attach to or enter new CD4 cells. For example, the replicative capacity (in vitro) of a virus resistant to lamivudine is decreased by over 50%. This (partly) explains why in cohort studies the rate of opportunistic infections and death among people on antiretroviral therapy, even if viral replication is not suppressed, is lower than untreated groups at comparable CD4 count and viral load.

Resistance to some drugs is conferred by a single mutation, so will develop very rapidly if viral replication occurs in the presence of the drug. Such drugs are best used in regimens that completely suppress viral replication. In others, multiple mutations are required and resistance develops over time, as new quasispecies with each advantageous mutation emerge sequentially. For some drugs, a mutation causing resistance to one drug will also cause cross-resistance to others of the same class. This occurs with available NNRTIs and with some protease and NRTI drugs.

Checklist: Terms used in HIV management

HAART:	Combinations of three or more antiretroviral drugs
Viral load:	Quantitative PCR for HIV viral RNA or bDNA
Viral suppression:	Viral load below the lower limit of detection of the available test
Undetectable:	Viral load below the lower limit of detection of the available test
Rebound[1]:	Viral load increase following an initial or sustained reduction
Blipping:	Brief increase in viral load above the limit of detection before becoming undetectable once more
Cross-resistance:	Genetic mutation making the virus resistant to one drug also confers resistance to others
Quasispecies:	Sub-populations of HIV in an individual with a particular genotype, sometimes conferring drug resistance

[1]'Failure' is another term used to describe an increase in viral load after suppression. It sometimes suggests that the patient has failed rather than the drugs, and is best avoided.

PRINCIPLES OF THERAPY

Combinations of two or more (usually three) antiretroviral drugs are given with the aim of reducing viral replication such that the plasma viral load drops below the limit of detection of the available assay. The most widely used assay in the UK detects 50 copies of virus per ml of plasma. In successful treatment, viral suppression should be achieved 12–16 weeks after starting therapy. The speed at which the viral load declines may affect the duration of suppression, and suppression is more durable when the viral load drops below 50 copies per ml than when it is between 50 and 400 copies per ml. There is no evidence of additional benefit in suppressing viral load below 5 copies per ml. At 1 year after starting a first HAART combination, viral suppression is maintained in 50–70% of patients in 'real' clinical cohorts or 80–90% of patients in some clinical trials. In the rest, viral suppression is not achieved, or occurs but then 'rebounds' because of adherence, absorption, pharmacological factors or pre-existing drug resistance. Over ensuing months and years, the proportion of the original cohort still maintaining viral suppression gradually reduces. If a second combination is given, including different drugs from the same class plus drugs from one or more new classes, again up to 60% of patients will achieve viral suppression to below 50 copies/ml. After a third drug combination, viral suppression is likely to be maintained in less than 50% of patients and a smaller reduction in viral load may be all that can be achieved. The choice of drugs used at each stage may affect the likelihood of successful therapy at the next: such 'sequencing' is the subject of a number of clinical trials.

Hence the appropriate management of antiretroviral therapy is different in different individuals and may change in each individual over time. The overall aim of therapy is to keep the viral load as low as possible for as long as possible, maintaining (or allowing recovery of) the CD4 count in order to:

- control symptoms due to HIV itself
- prevent opportunistic infections and malignancies.

These benefits must be balanced against:

- short- and long-term side effects
- interference with daily life
- removal of future therapeutic options.

The balance between these factors may be different in different situations; in the asymptomatic patient who is commencing therapy for the first time, even minor side effects may be unacceptable. In patients with a relatively low risk of disease progression, there may be benefit in waiting for newer and better tolerated or easier-to-take combinations (past experience would suggest this has been the case). In a patient who has taken multiple therapies and is left with few 'options', choices include combinations of up to seven different drugs (called mega-HAART), which may be difficult to take but give good viral control, or using a small number of drugs, with less effective viral control but better tolerability.

INITIATING THERAPY

The decision to initiate therapy in chronic HIV infection is a complex one. The patient must be fully and appropriately supported in deciding on the appropriate time to start and drugs used. In patients with AIDS, or with significant problematic symptoms of HIV, the potential benefit of treatment may be clear and the decision to commence therapy is straightforward. In other cases, the risk/benefit analysis is less obvious to both the patient and the treating doctor, and requires careful consideration. Some patients may wish to avoid therapy despite significant symptoms and severe immunosuppression. Informed decisions should be respected and the therapeutic relationship maintained in these cases. Guidelines on treatment must be interpreted in relation to the individual. Differences between UK and USA guidelines reflect the fact that the optimal timing of commencing therapy in asymptomatic individuals has not been defined. However, in most patients, treatment is indicated:

- in AIDS or other HIV related illness
- in asymptomatic patients with CD4 count of <200 cells/mm^3
- in some patients with CD4 count of 200–350 cells/mm^3.

In all cases, but particularly in the 'grey area' of CD4 count between 200 and 350 cells/mm^3, the decision to start can be affected by the rate of CD4 count decline, the viral load, the presence and controllability of non-AIDS symptoms and most importantly the social and psychological factors affecting the patients readiness for therapy. Figure 11.2 outlines some of the steps involved in deciding to commence therapy.

The drug combination recommended for first-line therapy in the UK is a combination of two NRTIs and one NNRTI. Other options that have been satisfactory in many patients include two NRTIs plus one or two protease inhibitors, or three NRTIs. As in other situations, information for patients should be pitched at an appropriate level. Commencing antiretroviral therapy is rarely an emergency and discussion can take place over three or more visits. Some patients will wish to fully research all possible options. In many patients, outlining the main potential pros and cons of two appropriate regimens after discussing the patient's priorities is useful. Factors to discuss include:

- the potential risk and benefits of immediate versus deferred therapy
- major short-term side effects and the probability of occurrence
- potential long-term side effects
- tablet number and tablet size
- dosage frequency
- possible implications for future therapeutic options (sequencing).

Side effects can be grouped into short-term self-limiting effects occurring on starting therapy, such as nausea with zidovudine, or dizziness with efavirenz. The symptoms of potentially dangerous acute side effects should be described (for example pancreatitis with didanosine, hypersensitivity to abacavir). Long-term side effects, discussed below, that may affect the patient's choice of drug should be discussed in detail (for example peripheral neuropathy with stavudine, didanosine or zalcitabine, lipodystrophy with PIs). Inevitably, the use of newly available drugs or combinations of drugs is based upon less accumulated evidence than those that have been available for some time. The easiest-to-take regimen may, therefore, be less proven in terms of efficacy and long-term side effects.

Case history

Tembi is a 28-year-old social worker who was diagnosed with HIV 3 years ago with a CD4 count of 340 cells/mm^3. She has had increasing problems with seborrhoeic dermatitis and her CD4 count has fallen to 224 cells/mm^3. She has been given literature and has discussed antiretroviral therapy with her doctor and an adherence support nurse in the clinic over the last three visits. Her main concerns are side effects that might expose her HIV status to her work colleagues: particularly rash and body shape changes. She works shifts and is keen to take her combination once-daily if possible.

She is considering the options of taking combivir twice-daily with efavirenz once in the evening, an option supported by a large body of evidence, or tenofovir together with efavirenz and either didanosine or lamivudine, which can be taken once daily, but is less well-proven.

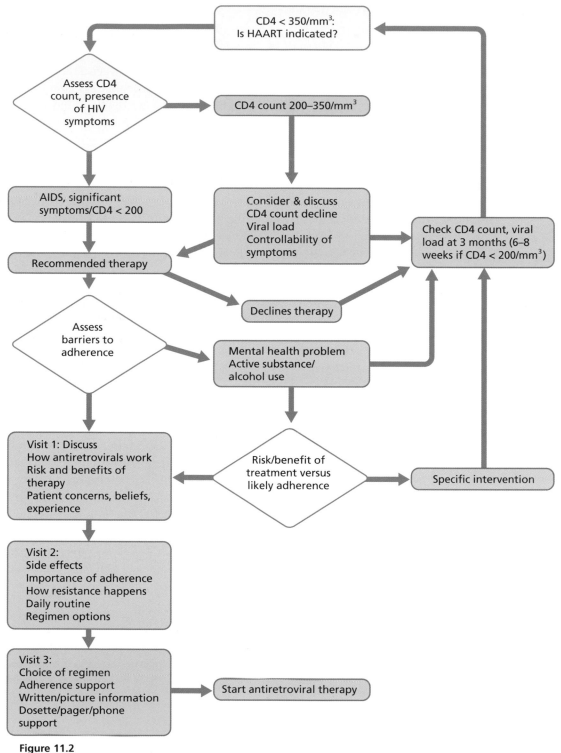

Figure 11.2
Commencing antiretroviral therapy

ANTIRETROVIRALS

NRTIs

NRTIs were the first antiretroviral drugs in clinical use. See Box 11.1 and Box 11.2 for details of available NRTIs. The majority of antiretroviral combinations (or regimens) in current use contain a 'backbone' of one or two nucleosides. The 'best' or most powerful combination has not been firmly established at the time of writing, but good evidence exists for the use of a thymidine analogue (AZT or D4T) in combination with either 3TC or DDI. The use of analogues of two different cellular nucleosides is recommended so that each drug is phosphorylated by a different cellular phosphorylase. Hence AZT and D4T are not used together because they are phosphorylated by the same intracellular thymidine kinase. The combination of D4T and DDI together may be more likely to cause peripheral neuropathy and is currently less popular. Regimens including three nucleoside drugs have been successfuly used together as initial therapy. A combination of three nucleosides is available and allows the prescription of one tablet twice daily (see Box 11.3). Evidence from comparative trials suggests that improved adherence may partly negate any deficit in drug efficacy, but three nucleoside regimens are probably not as effective as multi-class combinations, particularly in patients with high viral load (>100 000 copies/ml).

Clinical notes: Abacavir hypersensitivity reaction

- Occurs in 3–8% of patients
- Occasionally fatal
- Median time to onset 11 days (1 day to 6 weeks) from starting therapy
- Fever, urticarial or maculopapular rash
- Nausea, vomiting, diarrhoea
- Fatigue, malaise, musculoskeletal symptoms
- Occasionally respiratory symptoms
- May be confused with viral illness; rechallenge is most dangerous
- If abacavir stopped for any reason, restart under supervision
- Never rechallenge after hypersensitivity reaction.

Nucleotides

The first nucleotide licensed for treatment of HIV is tenofovir (Box 11.4). It is taken as a once-daily tablet with or just after food. Gastrointestinal side effects occur but are uncommon. Tenofovir is increasingly used as a component of a once-daily regimen. It interacts with didanosine, increasing plasma levels. The appropriate dose of DDI with tenofovir has not been determined at the time of writing. It is active against some viral strains resistant to AZT and 3TC.

NNRTIs

Combinations including two NRTIs and one NNRTI are the most widely prescribed 'first-line' regimen in the UK. The first two NNRTIs licensed in the UK were nevirapine and

Box 11.1: Nucleoside reverse transcriptase inhibitors

Photo	Drug	Abbreviation	Trade name	Dose
	Zidovudine	AZT	Retrovir	250 mg bd 300 mg bd
	Lamivudine	3TC	Epivir	150 mg twice-daily 300 mg once-daily
	Stavudine	D4T	Zerit	40 mg twice-daily (>60 kg) 30 mg twice-daily (<60 kg)
	Didanosine	DDI	Videx	200 mg twice-daily (>60 kg) 125 mg twice-daily (<60 kg)
	Didanosine		Videx EC	400 mg once-daily (>60 kg) 250 mg once-daily (<60 kg)
	Zalcitabine	DDC	Hivid	0.75 mg three times daily
	Abacavir		Ziagen	300 mg twice-daily 600 mg once-daily

Box 11.2: Notes on NRTIs

Drug	Notes
Zidovudine	First licensed NRTI: best established for use in preventing vertical transmission and post exposure prophylaxis Good CNS penetration: evidence for effect in AIDS dementia. Beneficial in HIV thrombocytopenia. Side effects include fatigue, malaise and nausea (often resolves after 4 weeks), anaemia due to bone marrow suppression (at 3 months after starting therapy, especially in advanced disease) and rarely, myopathy. Pigmentation of the nails and skin of the extremities may occur in people with black or brown skin
Lamivudine	A single mutation at site 184 confers resistance, so must be part of a maximally suppressive regimen Active against hepatitis B, so may be useful in co-infected patients but should not be discontinued (hepatic decompensation) Very well tolerated – short- and long-term adverse effects are rare
Stavudine	Few short-term adverse effects Long-term effects include peripheral neuropathy. Accumulating evidence that stavudine is more strongly implicated in the development of lipoatrophy than other NRTIs Effective against some AZT resistant viruses
Didanosine	Potent in combination with AZT. Long intracellular half-life. Gastrointestinal side effects (e.g. diarrhoea) are common with dispersible tablets and have affected adherence in some studies. They are less of a problem with chewable enteric coated tablets that also allow once-daily dosing. Should be taken 30 min before or 2 hours after food. Major side effect is pancreatitis, so avoid in those with past history or high alcohol intake
Zalcitabine	Effective but currently little used. Peripheral neuropathy and oral ulceration are the most significant side effects
Abacavir	Greater effect on viral load than other NRTIs when used alone in trials. Well tolerated, but hypersensitivity affects up to 9% of patients, manifesting as fever, rash, gastrointestinal or respiratory symptoms. May be fatal if drug continued, or if withdrawn and re-introduced

efavirenz. Their major limitation is the fact that a single mutation is sufficient to confer resistance to both drugs. They are probably most useful as components of a first antiretroviral regimen (see Box 11.5 and Box 11.6 for details). The use of two NNRTIs together has been little studied and is not widely prescribed. NNRTIs are not active against HIV 2. Both drugs are metabolized by the hepatic cytochrome p450 system in the liver and induce their own metabolism, as well as affecting the metabolism of other drugs.

The major side effects of nevirapine are rash and hepatitis (Fig. 11.3), usually but not always occurring in the first 6–8 weeks of treatment. Rash occurs in up to 17% of patients. The typical mild or moderate maculopapular rash can be treated with antihistamines until it resolves. The benefit of steroid treatment is unproven and prophylactic use to prevent rash has been shown to be ineffective. If rash is severe, the drug should be discontinued to avoid Stevens-Johnson syndrome. Disturbance of liver function is common (8–20%), especially in those co-infected with hepatitis B or C and liver function should be monitored every 2 weeks for the first 8 weeks of therapy.

Box 11.3: Combination nucleoside tablets

Photo	Drug	Contains	Trade name	Dose
	Combivir	Zidovudine 300 mg Lamivudine 150 mg	Combivir	One twice daily
	Trizivir	Zidovudine 300 mg Lamivudine 300 mg Abacavir 300 mg	Trizivir	One twice daily

Box 11.4: Nucleotide

Photo	Drug	Trade name	Dose
	Tenofovir	Viread	300 mg once daily

Clinically apparent hepatitis is rare, but potentially fatal: this has precluded the use of nevirapine as post exposure prophylaxis for HIV.

The major side effects of efavirenz are neuropsychiatric. Vivid dreams, dizziness and poor co-ordination are extremely common, reported in around 50% of patients. The impact of these symptoms may be reduced by taking the drug before bed. Major neuropsychiatric effects including depression are rare but sometimes become apparent only after prolonged treatment. A history of psychiatric or psychological disorder or substance use does not appear to increase the likelihood of side effects. Rash with efavirenz is less common than with nevirapine, affecting about 5% of patients, as is hepatitis. Delavirdine is licensed for use in the USA and Canada but is not recommended in the UK. It causes rash in up to 25% of patients.

Clinical notes: hepatotoxicity with nevirapine

Transaminases up to 5× basal level: interrupt treatment, reintroduce when transaminases return to baseline. If rapid increase occurs on re-introduction, stop permanently.

Transaminases over 2× basal level with symptoms of hypersensitivity (exanthema, fever, arthralgia, myalgia, adenopathy, eosinophilia): stop treatment permanently.

Transaminases over 2× basal level, no associated symptoms of hypersensitivity. Continue treatment under close supervision.

(From European Agency for the Evaluation of Medicinal Products Guidance)

Box 11.5: Non-nucleoside reverse transcriptase inhibitors

Photo	Drug	Abbreviation	Trade name	Dose
	Nevirapine	NVP	Viramune	200 mg twice daily 400 mg once daily
	Efavirenz	EFV	Sustiva	600 mg once daily on an empty stomach
	Delavirdine		Rescriptor	400 mg three times daily 600 mg twice daily

Protease inhibitors

Although HAART regimens that do not include protease inhibitor (PI) drugs have been used with increasing confidence in recent years, the best evidence for the use of antiretrovirals to prevent AIDS defining illness or death applies to combinations including a protease inhibitor (Box 11.7 and Box 11.8). Consequently, some clinicians consider a protease inhibitor-containing regimen to be preferable in patients with advanced disease or with AIDS at diagnosis. Protease inhibitor-containing regimens may also be preferable

Box 11.6: Notes on NNRTIs

Drug	Notes
Nevirapine	Start at 200 mg once daily for 2 weeks, then increase to therapeutic dose if no rash. Monitor LFTs two weekly. Abnormal LFTs do not necessitate discontinuation, but 1–5% of patients do have to discontinue due to biochemical or clinical hepatitis. Interacts with most PIs (lowering levels). Reduces methadone levels.
Efavirenz	Several cohort studies suggest efavirenz may be more likely to achieve and maintain viral suppression than nevirapine. A randomized controlled trial did not support this finding. Half-life is over 40 hours, so is regarded as 'forgiving' of late or missed doses. Neuropsychiatric side effects may be severe but usually settle after the first 2–4 weeks. Depression, suicidal ideation and vague depersonalization symptoms are sometimes reported after months on therapy. Plasma levels are significantly lower if taken without food, so may reduce side effects. TDM and dose reduction may also be useful. Both induces and inhibits cytochrome p450 system, so variable interactions with other drugs.

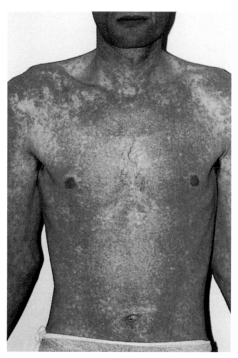

Figure 11.3
Nevirapine rash

in patients who have previously been exposed to NRTIs as mono or dual therapy. They are also usually indicated in 'second-line' and subsequent regimens following viral rebound on an initial regimen containing an NNRTI. The major disadvantages of PIs have been short half-lives, requiring multiple daily doses, a high frequency of gastrointestinal side effects and long-term changes in body morphology and lipid metabolism. Interactions with other drugs are also common, which sometimes complicates the treatment of opportunistic infections and other conditions. Some PIs also

Box 11.7: Protease inhibitors

Photo	Drug	Abbreviation	Trade name	Dose[1]
	Ritonavir	RTV	Norvir	RTV 600 mg twice daily RTV 400 mg twice daily with SQV or IDV RTV 100 mg twice daily or RTV 200 mg once daily as a 'booster' for other proteases
	Saquinavir Hard gel capsules	SQV (HGC)	Invirase	SQV 400 mg twice daily with RTV 400 mg twice daily SQV1000 mg twice daily with RTV 100 mg twice daily
	Soft gel capsules	SQV (SGC)	Fortovase	SQV 1200 mg three times daily with food (not as single PI)
	Indinavir	IDV	Crixivan	IDV 800 mg three times daily 2 hours after food or with low fat meal IDV 800 mg twice daily with RTV 100 mg twice daily, no food restriction (high incidence renal stones)
	Nelfinavir	NFV	Viracept	NFV 750 mg three times daily NFV 1250 mg twice daily

Box 11.7: Protease inhibitors (Cont'd)

Photo	Drug	Abbreviation	Trade name	Dose[1]
	Lopinavir/ritonavir	LPV/r	Kaletra	LPV/RTV 400 mg/100 mg (three capsules) twice daily with food
	Amprenavir	APV	Agenerase	AMP 1200 mg twice daily AMP 600 mg twice daily with RTV 100 mg twice daily AMP 1200 mg once daily with RTV 200 mg once daily
	Fos-amprenavir[2]	Fos-APV	Telzir	Fos-APV 1400 mg once daily with ritonavir 100 mg once daily
	Atazanavir[2]	ATZ		ATZ 400 mg once daily

[1]Includes licensed and unlicensed dosages
[2]Not licensed in Europe at mid 2003. Dosages from expanded access/named patient programmes

Box 11.8: Notes on PIs

Drug	Notes
Ritonavir	Take 2 hours apart from didanosine. High incidence of GI side effects, particularly diarrhoea. Lipid abnormalities (especially triglycerides). Circumoral and peripheral paraesthesia. Potent inhibitor of cytochrome p450: multiple drug interactions. Start on lower dose and escalate if used alone: 300 mg bd for 2 days, 400 mg bd for 3 days, 500 mg bd for 7 days, then full dose.
Saquinavir	HGC should be given only with RTV. Side effects: diarrhoea, nausea and abdominal pain occur.
Indinavir	Crystallizes in the urinary tract. Renal tract stones (flank pain, haematuria) occur in 4% or more if boosted with ritonavir. High fluid intake (>1.5 L per day) required and beware dehydration if travel, diarrhoea or vomiting. Side effects: dry skin, nail changes and hair loss occur.

Box 11.8: Notes on PIs (Cont'd)

Drug	Notes
Nelfinavir	Has been used as a 'first-line' protease drug because mutations conferring resistance to nelfinavir do not usually cause resistance to other proteases. Side effect: diarrhoea in 60%.
Lopinavir/ritonavir	Evidence of better antiviral effect than single PI (nelfinavir). Side effects as ritonavir (especially lipid abnormalities). Some activity against viruses resistant to other PIs.
Amprenavir	High pill burden if given alone (8 capsules twice daily). Not approved as first-line therapy because less effective than other PIs or efavirenz. Side effects: diarrhoea, nausea, especially initially.
Fos-amprenavir	Prodrug of amprenavir with a lower pill burden.
Atazanavir	Appears to have less adverse effects on serum lipids than other PIs. Hyperbilirubinaemia in up to 30%, rarely, jaundice. Resistance may not confer resistance to other proteases.

inhibit their own metabolism and that of other protease drugs by the cytochrome p450 system. When two (or more) are taken together, this inhibition may improve the pharmacokinetic profile such that doses can be given once or twice daily and without dietary restrictions. This increases the attractiveness of PI containing regimens as first-line therapy. Ritonavir appears to have this effect at subtherapeutic doses as low as 100 mg twice daily, although, unfortunately, from the limited evidence currently available its gastrointestinal side effects and effects on metabolism may occur even at this dose.

Fusion inhibitors

Enfuvirtide (T20) was the first drug to be developed that inhibits the fusion of the viral membrane of HIV 1 with the CD4 cell membrane. It causes a significant drop in viral load when used alone in patients who have been exposed to all other available antiretroviral drugs. It is given by subcutaneous injection and has been used principally in salvage therapy. Other fusion inhibitors are under development.

ADVERSE EFFECTS OF HAART

The long-term adverse effects associated with HAART toxicity are major factors affecting patient safety and quality of life (Box 11.9). Some of these toxicities are regarded as 'class effects', and are associated to a variable extent with all drugs with a common mechanism of action. Toxicities of both NRTIs and PIs may both contribute to the syndrome of lipodystrophy.

Lactic acidosis

Some toxicities of nucleoside drugs (NRTIs) may be related to adverse effects on cellular mitochondria. NRTIs have minimal inhibitory effect on human DNA polymerase alpha, the enzyme responsible for nuclear DNA replication. However, human mitochondrial DNA is replicated by DNA polymerase gamma, which is inhibited by NRTIs to a variable extent. Mitochondrial DNA depletion and the resultant disorder of cellular oxidative

Box 11.9: Toxicities associated with HAART

	Complication	Intervention
Lipid changes: Hypercholesterolaemia Raised serum LDL Raised triglycerides	Pancreatitis (triglycerides) ? Increased atherosclerosis ? Increased cardiac risk ? Increased CVA risk	Stop PIs (change to ABC or NVP may improve lipid profiles) Manage other risk factors as in HIV uninfected (exercise, BP, smoking) Dietary modification Statins (pravastatin 1st choice) Fibrates
Lipodystrophy	Stigmatisation	Stop PIs, D4T (prevent progression)
Lipoatrophy	Low self-esteem Depression Psychosexual disorder	Cosmetic surgery
Insulin resistance	Glucose intolerance Exacerbation of pre-existing diabetes mellitus New-onset diabetes mellitus Increased cardiovascular risk	Oral hypoglycaemic and/or stop PIs. Reversibility on stopping not clear
Osteopenia Osteoporosis	Fractures	No evidence for routine screening by DEXA scan but consider other risk factors Treatment as in HIV uninfected

phosphorlation is suggested (but not proven) to underly many of the side effects of NRTIs:

- Hyperlactataemia and lactic acidosis
- Peripheral neuropathy
- Pancreatitis
- Lipoatrophy (fat wasting)
- Myopathy
- Bone marrow suppression.

Moderate hyperlactataemia (uncuffed venous serum lactate 2.5–5 mmol/l) occurs in over 10% of those on therapy and does not predict the occurrence of lactic acidosis. Routine monitoring of serum lactate is not recommended for people on HAART. Lactic acidosis is fortunately rare but often fatal. Treatment is essentially supportive. Symptoms are non-

Clinical notes: diagnosis of lactic acidosis

Symptoms	Investigation
Nausea	Uncuffed serum lactate > 5 mmol/l
Vomiting	pH < 7.35
Weight loss	Anion gap $((Na+K - (Cl+CO_2))>18$
Abdominal distension	Abnormal LFTs
Weakness	
Dyspnoea	
Myalgia	

specific and variable so all patients on NRTIs with unexplained gastrointestinal symptoms, fatigue, weight loss or weakness should be investigated for lactic acidosis.

Dyslipidaemia and lipodystrophy

Lipid abnormalities are associated with the use of most, but not all PIs and to a lesser degree with efavirenz. Serum dislipidaemia associated with PI use is often associated with changes in body shape termed lipodystrophy, with increases in intra-abdominal fat, breast enlargement and cervical fat pads ('buffalo hump') accompanied by wasting of the buccal and temporal fat pads and the subcutaneous fat of the limbs. Although changes in serum lipids, particularly triglycerides, occur when ritonavir is given to healthy volunteers, it appears that other complex metabolic abnormalities and body shape changes that occur with HAART involve synergistic effects of PIs, NRTIs and perhaps the indirect effects of reducing HIV replication and the resultant immune recovery. The fat wasting component of the syndrome (lipoatrophy) has been observed in those treated with NRTIs alone and may be more strongly associated with stavudine (Fig. 11.4). Lipodystrophy has been reported in 30–85% of those taking HAART and significantly affects quality of life. It

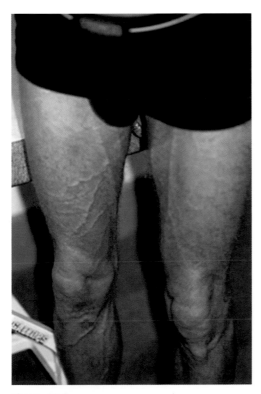

Figure 11.4
Peripheral lipoatrophy

identifies the individual among peers as HIV positive and has been clearly associated with loss of self-esteem and depression. Other concerns relating to dislipidaemia include the likelihood of increased atherosclerotic complications with HAART. Options for intervention in those affected include exercise, dietary modification, lipid-lowering agents and, where possible, changing antiretroviral therapy to include drugs less strongly implicated with the problem. Changing to a 'PI sparing' regimen often improves lipid profiles but the evidence suggests that any significant improvement in lipodystrophy is likely to take many years. Plastic surgery procedures can reduce the cosmetic impact of local lipomatosis and facial lipoatrophy.

Other metabolic effects

Hyperglycaemia with insulin resistance and new onset diabetes mellitus occur in association with PI use. Routine glucose tolerance tests are not indicated but some clinicians perform a 3–12 monthly fasting glucose level. Reductions in bone-mineral density seem to be more common in people taking PIs than other HIV infected individuals.

ADHERENCE

The level of adherence to HAART is closely associated with the likelihood of viral suppression and is largely responsible for the difference in reported outcomes between patients in clinical trials and those in the clinic setting. Over 95% of doses must be taken correctly to achieve satisfactory viral suppression. Supporting and maintaining adherence is the cornerstone of HIV management and as adherence can vary in the same person over time (usually deteriorating), adherence should be addressed at regular outpatient appointments. A team approach to support is required; this may involve doctor, pharmacist, psychologist, nursing staff, specialist adherence staff, voluntary sector workers, other patient group representatives or buddies. Adherence is improved when patients are involved in decisions regarding therapy and understand the reason for treatment and the choice of drugs. Hence, perhaps the most important factor in successful therapy is that it should start only when the patient is ready. Health workers, particularly doctors are particularly poor at predicting adherence and there is little evidence to suggest that particular groups (for example ex-drug users) are less likely to adhere. Some factors known to affect adherence are:

- Health beliefs
- Current alcohol/drug use
- Depression
- Understanding therapy
- Doctor–patient relationship
- Dosage frequency
- Side effects.

Demographic factors such as race, age, gender, social class and educational level are not consistently associated with adherence. Box 11.10 outlines some of the interventions to consider to improve adherence.

Box 11.10: Addressing adherence

Factor	Intervention
Understanding and health beliefs	Discuss mechanism of drug resistance and importance of adherence prior to commencement. Explore feared side-effects, problems and choose regimen appropriately. Give written (or picture) information, including pill charts or calendars
Side effects	Discuss and anticipate possible side effects. Provide easy access to, or prophylactic symptom relief (e.g. loperamide with ritonavir). Be prepared to change regimen early if side effects severe
Practical barriers	Run through daily/weekly routine. Explore times when difficulties may arise (travel, weekends). Avoid changing routine to suit regimen if possible. Explore concern re. disclosure of status through medication (colleagues, relatives). Ensure access to repeat prescription. Consider 'fall-back' supply for patient to keep in reserve
Forgetfulness	Commonest stated reason for missed doses. Try alarm watch or prompt on mobile phone. Relative/friend or buddy to prompt, especially in the first few weeks. Dosette box. Trial run with multivitamin pills or sweets
Regimen factors	Once or twice daily regimens are better adhered to than 3 or 4 times a day. Pill burden may also affect adherence. Avoid/accommodate food restrictions. Acceptability of the regimen to the patient and their lifestyle usually outweighs other factors
Maintenance	Reassess social and lifestyle factors regularly. Address adherence at every visit. Stay alert to development of depression or new side effects

CHANGING THERAPY

The need to change antiretroviral therapy will present itself in most (if not all) patients eventually. In patients in whom therapy has previously been very successful, either in terms of symptom relief or surrogate markers or both, the realization that therapy has 'stopped working' after a prolonged period of complete viral suppression can have great impact. This can be a stressful and difficult time for many patients. Issues such as side effects and adherence must be re-addressed. Worries about illness and lifespan may be revisited and adequate support should be offered. The indications for change include:

1. *Inadequate suppression of viral load.* The viral load has not fallen to below the limit of detection of the available test by 24 weeks.
2. *Viral load rebound.* Having been undetectable for some time (months or years), the viral load has risen.
3. *Fall in CD4 count.* A patient who has continued on therapy with a detectable viral load is experiencing a fall in CD4 count to a level carrying an increased risk of complications.
4. *New symptoms or opportunistic infection.*
5. *Intolerable side effects.*
6. *Treatment fatigue.* A patient who started therapy when symptomatic and has experienced good immune recovery may wish to stop therapy or change to an easier to take regimen.

7. *Change in risk/benefit ratio.* An improvement in immune status and reduction in HIV-related risk, or a new clinical event has made the risks associated with therapy unacceptable (for example, a myocardial infarct occurring in a hypercholesterolaemic patient taking PIs).

In most cases change will include all the drugs in a HAART regimen. Exceptions include treatment intensification – the addition of an extra drug to an existing regimen. This is usually done when the viral load has failed to become undetectable in the first few months of therapy. Figure 11.5 outlines the monitoring and interventions possible in the months following initiation of a first or second therapeutic regimen. The decision to change therapy in a patient on established treatment depends upon:

- current clinical status
- clinical status at the time of diagnosis
- previous and current adherence
- acceptability of the current regimen
- side effects of the current compared to a future regimen
- viral load
- current CD4 count
- CD4 count at initiation of treatment
- current antiretrovirals
- resistance test data
- previous antiviral exposure
- currently available options
- future treatment options.

Thresholds for regarding surrogate markers as indicative of the need for change are not precisely defined. In patients taking their first or second HAART combination, treatment may be changed as soon as an increase in viral load above the limit of detection is confirmed by at least one further sample. This is done with the aim of reducing the development of further mutations that might compromise the effectiveness of future treatment options. In others, a rise in viral load to several thousand copies/ml in an asymptomatic patient with no side effects from their current drugs may provoke no change. In those who have been exposed to multiple drug combinations the correct course of action is not clearly defined. So-called 'salvage therapy' might include some new drugs and drugs to which the patient has previously been exposed. The tolerability of the regimen, particularly in the case of 'mega-HAART' therapy, then becomes a major issue. Decisions to change, in people who have relatively few treatment options remaining, are also influenced by the fact that the probability of a new clinical event in someone taking therapy and with a viral load of less than 5000 copies/ml is low. Before contemplating changing treatment, it is important to consider in every case the reasons why current therapy is not achieving the desired outcome. These might include:

- adherence
- viral resistance to drugs
- pharmacokinetic factors (food restrictions, drug interactions, individual variations in drug handling).

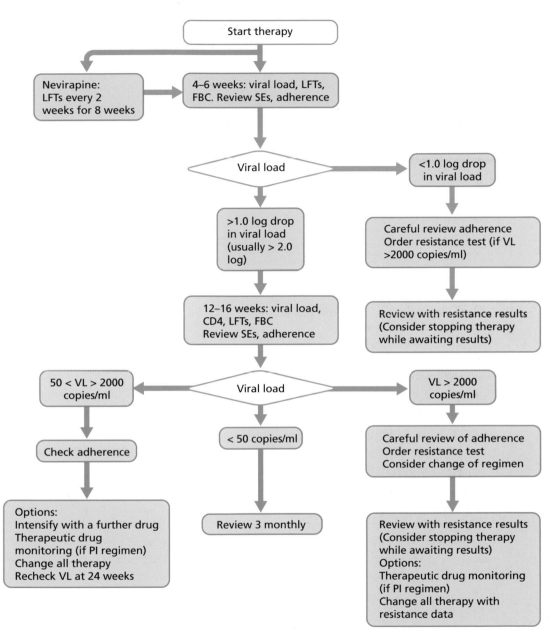

Figure 11.5
Follow-up after commencing antiretroviral therapy

These factors should be addressed individually. Adherence should be discussed in detail. In some cases an improvement in adherence is sufficient to successfully suppress the viral load once more. Pharmacokinetic factors can be assessed by the use of therapeutic drug monitoring and viral resistance can be investigated using genotypic and phenotypic resistance testing.

RESISTANCE TESTS

Resistance tests are of two main types, the genotypic test and the phenotypic test.

Genotypic tests

Genotypic tests amplify the viral genome using PCR and either use oligonucleotide probes to sample relevant sections of the genome, identifying genetic mutations known from previous laboratory studies to be associated with resistance to particular drugs, or sequence the sections of the genome encoding the relevant enzymes. Genotypic tests are relatively inexpensive and quick to perform.

Phenotypic tests

Phenotypic tests involve culture of a laboratory clone of HIV containing reverse transcriptase and protease genes from the patient's virus in the presence of the drug. The ability of the drug to inhibit viral replication is measured compared to a reference virus. Phenotypic tests are considerably more time consuming and expensive to perform, but may reflect more accurately the in-vivo effect of resistance mutations on drug response.

A widely used refinement of genotypic testing involves matching the genotype of the sample to a massive database of phenotypic data to predict the likely resistance profile of the viral strain. Interpretation of resistance test data is highly complex and evolves rapidly. A few of the commonly encountered resistance mutations are included in Box 11.11. Limitations of resistance tests include the following:

- They are usually successful only if the viral load is greater than 2000 copies/ml
- They don't detect minority viral quasispecies, so usually detect only mutations conferring resistance to drugs being taken at the time the sample was obtained.

THERAPEUTIC DRUG MONITORING

There is wide variation in individual absorption of protease inhibitors. Measurement of plasma levels can be used to inform dose adjustment, either to ensure that levels are adequate for viral suppression, or to avoid side effects. These issues may be less important with the use of dual-PI regimens. Plasma levels of efavirenz can also be quantified, but the levels of NRTIs in plasma do not correlate with the intracellular level and are not routinely measured.

Box 11.11: Examples of HIV resistance mutations

Mutations at codons	May confer viral resistance to:
41, 67, 210, 215, 219	AZT, D4T
184	3TC
69 (insertion), 151	All NRTIs
103, 181	NNRTIs
82, 84, 90	PIs

Further Reading

Bell C, Matthews GV, Nelson MR. Non-nucleoside reverse transcriptase inhibitors – an overview. Int Jour STD & AIDS 2003; 14: 71–77.

BHIVA Writing Committee on behalf of the BHIVA Executive Committee. British HIV Association guidelines for the treatment of HIV-infected adults with antiretroviral therapy. HIV Med 2001; 2: 276–313.

Centers for Disease Control and Prevention. Guidelines for using antiretroviral agents among HIV-infected adults and adolescents. Ann Intern Med 2002; 137: 38.

Egger M, May M, Chene G, et al. Prognosis of HIV-1 infected patients starting highly active antiretroviral therapy: a collaborative analysis of prospective studies. Lancet 2002; 360: 119–129.

Gazzard B. Scientific evidence and expert clinical opinion for the institution of salvage therapy. In: Gazzard BG, Johnson M, Miles A (eds). The effective management of HIV/AIDS. London; Aesculapius Medical Press: 2001.

Piscitelli SC, Gallicano KD. Interactions among drugs for HIV and opportunistic infections. N Eng J Med 2001; 344: 984–996.

SELF-ASSESSMENT

Laurence is a 36-year-old barman. He was diagnosed HIV positive 4 years ago when his CD4 count was 320 cells/mm^3. He attended the clinic infrequently, missing several appointments. There was a gap of a year before his last attendance, 2 weeks ago, when he had bloods taken. He has lost a little weight, is having night sweats and feels 'pretty low'. He returns to the clinic to discuss the results. His CD4 count is 159 cells/mm^3, viral load 79 000 copies per ml (RT-PCR).

a) What is his estimated risk of developing AIDS within 3 years without therapy?
b) Suggest three factors from what you already know that should be considered with regard to his adherence, before starting therapy.
c) What practical steps could you take to help support adherence?
d) After discussing the options, he decides not to take antiretrovirals. What do you do?

Answers
a) 85.5% (see Fig. 9.3, Ch. 9).
b) *Consider his knowledge of therapy.* What are his feelings about medical care and taking medicines in general? Does he know anyone who is taking antiretroviral therapy? What drugs and side effects has he heard of, if any? What potential side effects concern him? Does he feel that now is the time to start?
Psychological and social factors. What is happening in his life just now that might affect his mental state? Are things stable or changing? Consider work, accommodation, finances, relationships, drug and alcohol use. Explore 'feeling low'. Does this relate to his physical symptoms or are there symptoms of a depressive illness? How does he feel about the prospect of starting therapy? What does it mean to him?
Practical barriers. Explore his intermittent attendance at clinics. What stops him attending appointments? Can anything be done to help with this? Will he be able to collect prescriptions regularly? Run through his daily/weekly routine. What hours does he work? Does he work shifts? What does he do when not working? Who knows about his diagnosis?
c) The regimen chosen may be important: consider whether a once daily regimen might be helpful (particularly if he works shifts). Pill number may be an issue, but is probably less important. Most first-line regimens in current use do not have food restrictions, so this should not be a problem.
Support from professionals (nurse, pharmacist, adherence support worker) or the voluntary sector may be available. The support of a partner, relative or friend might help. A dosette box may be useful. A pager or alarm watch might avoid missed doses. Telephone support from the clinic or voluntary sector may be possible.
d) Encourage him to attend the clinic a little more regularly: at least within 3 months and preferably sooner. Discuss taking prophylaxis against PCP and commence immediately if he agrees. Give treatment for any other minor symptoms such as skin problems. Refer to psychological or psychiatric services if indicated. Give information on access to care if he becomes unwell. Explore the reasons for his decision for further discussion in future. Book an early review appointment.

Appendix: Treatment of sexually transmitted infections in pregnancy

Sexually transmitted infections in pregnancy have several possible adverse effects including:

- spontaneous abortion or intrauterine death
- foetal abnormality due to in-utero transmission
- premature rupture of membranes, premature labour and low-birth weight
- neonatal complications due to intrapartum transmission
- teratogenic effects of therapeutic drugs
- complications or increased severity of maternal illness during pregnancy.

Only those factors affecting the immediate outpatient management of a pregnant woman diagnosed with STI are covered here. Further details and management of the affected neonate are not included.

Box A1: Bacterial sexually transmitted infections in pregnancy

Transmission, maternal and neonatal effects	Management of maternal infection
Neisseria gonorrhoeae Transmission: intrapartum Neonate: ophthalmia neonatorum, septicaemia, arthritis	As non-pregnant woman. Avoid quinolones and tetracyclines Ceftriaxone 250 mg i.m. single dose or spectinomycin 2 g i.m. single dose
Chlamydia trachomatis Transmission: effects on endometrium and membranes, in-utero transmission may be possible. Intrapartum transmission common. Maternal effects: early spontaneous abortion (?). Premature rupture of membranes. Neonate: ophthalmia neonatorum in 75%, pneumonia in 20% of infants born to infected mothers.	Amoxycillin 250 mg three times daily for a week or erythromycin 500 mg twice daily for a week (erythromycin is more efficacious but less well tolerated). Azithromycin 1 g single dose is not licensed in pregnancy but has been widely used without adverse effect. Perform test-of-cure.

Box A1: (Cont'd) Bacterial sexually transmitted infections in pregnancy

Transmission, maternal and neonatal effects	Management of maternal infection
Syphilis	Penicillin regimens as in non-pregnant patients. If history of penicillin allergy, skin testing to detect hypersensitivity and inpatient desensitization regimen. Check VDRL through pregnancy and treat neonate if any doubt about regimen, compliance or response to therapy, or if treated in last 4 weeks. Some recommend retreatment in pregnancy, even if history of successful treatment.
Transmission: in-utero. In the first year after acquiring syphilis, 90% chance of transmission to the foetus. Neonatal effects: 30% of foetuses will be stillborn without treatment and 14% if the mother is treated. Most live born foetuses appear well. When a few months old, 40% develop symptoms of early syphilis including skin rashes, rhinitis and bony abnormalities. Late disease includes interstitial keratitis and bony and neurological abnormalities that appear from late childhood until well into adulthood.	

Box A2: Trichomonas vaginalis *and bacterial vaginosis in pregnancy*

Transmission, maternal and neonatal effects	Management of maternal infection
Trichomonas vaginalis	
Transmission: intrapartum Maternal effects: possibly prematurity Neonatal effects: vulvovaginitis	As non-pregnant woman, but avoid single-dose metronidazole Metronidazole 400 mg twice daily for 7 days from second trimester onwards
Bacterial vaginosis	
Transmission: no Maternal effects: premature rupture of membranes and preterm birth (see Ch. 3)	As non-pregnant woman, but avoid single dose metronidazole Metronidazole 400 mg twice daily for 7 days from second trimester onwards

Box A3: Viral sexually transmitted infections in pregnancy

Transmission, maternal and neonatal effects	Management of maternal infection
Genital warts Transmission: intrapartum (<1%) Maternal effects: warts may first appear or worsen during pregnancy. Neonatal effects: laryngeal papillomatosis in children born to women with and without warts. Anogenital warts in neonates very rare.	Spontaneous regression post delivery is common – reassure. Use cryotherapy if treatment desired. Neither treatment nor caesarean section known to reduce risk of HPV transmission.
Herpes simplex virus Transmission: intrapartum (1.7/100 000 live births UK). Primary infection 40% transmission, recurrent infection <8%. Maternal effects: primary infection in early pregnancy – spontaneous abortion. Disseminated herpes in mother very rare. Neonatal effects: primary infection in third trimester – herpes neonatorum. Severe systemic illness fatal without treatment.	Aciclovir unlicensed in pregnancy but widely used in standard doses. Treat on clinical grounds as in non-pregnant patients. Elective caesarean section (ECS) at term if primary genital herpes in last 6 weeks of pregnancy. ECS in recurrent herpes at term unproven. Use of aciclovir to suppress recurrence at term unproven. Prevention: if partner has history of herpes, mother does not, advise condom use during pregnancy, avoid sex if symptomatic. Use of type-specific serology to determine seroconcordance/discordance possible.

Box A4: Blood-borne virus infections in pregnancy

Transmission, maternal and neonatal effects	Interventions to reduce transmission
HIV Transmission: 15–25% in non-breastfeeding populations. Up to 40% with breastfeeding. Higher transmission if low CD4, high VL, prolonged rupture of membranes, prematurity. Maternal effects: no increase in progression unless advanced disease.	Transmission with AZT alone (maternal, during labour and neonate for 6 weeks) is 7%, AZT + 3TC; 2.5%, HAART; 1–2%. Additional benefit of elective caesarean section if mother on successful HAART is unproven, complications of ECS higher in HIV-positive women. Planned pregnancy in woman on therapy; consider stopping for first trimester, avoid efavirenz. If CD4 >350 cells/mm^3, not on therapy, start HAART (e.g. AZT, 3TC, NVP) at 20–24 weeks, aim for viral load <50 copies/ml at delivery. Otherwise treat according to maternal requirements. VL<50 does not guarantee zero transmission. Avoid breastfeeding.
Hepatitis B Transmission: intrapartum and postnatal. Possibly intrauterine. 90% transmission if HBeAg positive, 10% if HBsAg positive, HBeAg negative. Neonatal effects: acute hepatitis B, 90% develop chronic infection.	Infant: hepatitis B vaccination within 12 hours of birth with hepatitis B immunoglobulin.
Hepatitis C Transmission: 5–6% if hepatitis C alone. Greater if co-infection with HIV.	Caesarean section may reduce transmission – unproven.

281

Index